Venereology
in Practice

Venereology in Practice

The Sexually Committed Diseases

BY

NEILS HJORTH, M.D.

Professor of Dermatology, The University Hospital
of Gentofte, Copenhagen, Denmark

AND

HENNING SCHMIDT, M.D.

Chief Physician, Professor of Dermatology,
The University Hospital of Odense, Denmark

English Language Edition Edited by

HOWARD I. MAIBACH, M.D.

Professor of Dermatology
University of California School of Medicine
San Francisco, California

Year Book Medical Publishers, Inc.
CHICAGO · LONDON

Library of Congress Cataloging in Publication Data
Hjorth, Niels.
  Venereology in practice.
  Translation of Praktisk venerologi.
  Includes index.
  1. Venereal diseases. I. Schmidt, Henning,
1922–   joint author. II. Maibach, Howard I.
III. Title. [DNLM: 1. Venereal diseases.
WC140 H677p]
RC200.2.H5813   616.9'51   79-10995
ISBN 0-8151-5728-2

Copyright © 1979 by Year Book Medical Publishers, Inc.

This book is an authorized translation from the original Danish edition published and copyrighted © 1976 by Munksgaard A.S., Copenhagen, Denmark. Title of the original Danish Edition: Praktisk venerologi.

The color illustrations have been made by clinical photographers from the Dermatology Departments at The Finsen Institute, The University Hospital of Gentofte, The Municipal Hospital of Copenhagen, The Marselisborg Hospital, and The University Hospital of Odense. A few illustrations have kindly been loaned by Professor Hans Rorsman, Lund, and Dr. Niels Rosman, Hillerød.

Contents

Introduction 5
Examination of the patient with venereal disease 8
   Examination of Men 8
   Examination of Women 9
Gonorrhea 11
   Gonorrhea in Men 12
   Gonorrhea in Women 13
   Extragenital Gonorrhea 15
   Diagnosis 17
   Treatment 21
Nongonococcal urethritis 26
   Chlamydia Trachomatis Infection . . . 27
   Ureaplasma (Mycoplasma) 29
   Bacterial NGU
       and Allied Genital Infections . . . 30
   Streptococci Group B 30
   Treatment 31
Reiter's Syndrome 32
Trichomoniasis 34
Candidiasis 36
Herpes Progenitalis 38
Syphilis 42
   Etiology 42
   Clinical Features 43
   Microscopic Diagnosis 48
   Serologic Diagnosis 49
   Treatment 53
Lymphogranuloma Venereum 57
Chancroid 59
Scabies 61
Pubic Lice 63
Condylomata Acuminata 65
Molluscum Contagiosum 68
Balanitis 69

Synergistic gangrene	71
Hepatitis	72
Other Skin Diseases of the Genitalia	73
Venerophobia	74
Plates	75
Index	99

Introduction

Definition For some sexually transmitted diseases the etiology is known; for others it is not. A common characteristic is that intimate contact is required for them to be communicated from one person to another. Many other diseases, such as influenza, hepatitis, tonsillitis and others, can be communicated by intimate contact; however, these can be transmitted by other means as well. The sexually transmitted diseases are reviewed here as thoroughly as their present prevalences warrant. The text is intended to provide the amount of knowledge reasonably expected of medical students and practicing physicians.

In addition to the "usual" diseases (syphilis, gonorrhea, chancroid and lymphogranuloma venereum) others include trichomoniases, crabs, scabies, herpes and the so-called nongonorrheic urethritis. There are reliable clinical symptoms of urethritis, but its etiology varies. Furthermore, this disease group includes molluscum contagiosum, balanitis, candidiasis and condylomata acuminata.

Chancroid and lymphogranuloma venereum are uncommon.

These diseases are characteristic in that they are located on the mucous membranes of the urogenital area, the skin of the genital organs and around the pubic hair. Unusual complications or rare clinical manifestations encountered by the venereologist only occasionally have been excluded.

Incidence In most countries, there is adequate information on the incidence of syphilis, gonorrhea, lymphogranuloma venereum, chancroid and scabies. Reasonably accurate statistics reflect the epidemiology of these diseases.

The frequency of the sexually transmitted diseases varies from one period of time to another. Despite the use of fully effective treatment procedures, it has not been possible to eliminate these diseases and they even increased significantly during the 1960s. In Denmark, after oral contraceptives became generally available in 1966, a significant increase was noted subsequently, whereas in Sweden, the increase had already occurred around 1960. The current increase cannot be entirely explained by the introduction of oral contraception. Social and economic conditions influence the incidence of the disease, as demonstrated by the increased incidence during wars, social unrest and economic booms (more alcoholism, more tourism). The influence exerted by these various factors is not certain. Likewise, the incidence within various social groups, for example, among students, foreign workers and other social categories, has not been adequately investigated.

Legislation about venereal disease The attitude toward sexually transmitted diseases has changed considerably over the years, partly because the etiology of most infectious diseases is now known and effective therapy is available. The legislation has also been influenced by the fact that the morally condemning attitude that prevailed in the past has been replaced by a more liberal view.

Treatment procedure A physician visited by a patient believed to have contracted a venereal disease has the following possible courses of action.

He may refer the patient to a specialist or public clinic and simultaneously inform these about the patient's data; or he may examine and treat the patient and, furthermore, call in for examination and any necessary treatment all the persons reported to have had sexual contact with the patient.

Tracing the source of contamination

Tracing the source of infection is of critical importance. A thorough knowledge of the patient's sexual contacts is essential in order to provide examination and, if necessary, treatment to all individuals involved, which is the only chance to carry on an even relatively effective fight against venereal disease. It is important to explain to the patient why such information is necessary.

Examination of the Patient with Venereal Disease

In examining the patient who has either come voluntarily for examination or has been referred because of suspicion of having a sexually transmitted disease, it is best to proceed in systematic fashion. The examination begins with the patient's history, which includes symptoms and date of exposure. At the same time, previous symptoms of identical or similar nature must be tracked down, as well as any previous sexually transmitted diseases that have run their course.

Examination of Men

Genital examination

During the examination of men, the urethral meatus is inspected and the skin and mucous membranes of the genitals are examined for ulcerations and condylomas. A secretion sample is then taken from the urethra (Fig. 1) for direct microscopic examination and culture for gonococci; trichomoniasis and, possibly, fungus investigations or ordinary bacteriologic cultures are also performed. After this, the epididymis and the contents of the scrotum are palpated to detect swelling and soreness. The lymph nodes in the groin, if palpable, are examined for any enlargement; their consistency, soreness and the appearance of the overlying skin are noted. Attention is paid to whether the lymph nodes are matted and adherent to the skin or the underlying tissue. Pubic hairs are examined for the presence of parasites.

Anal examination The anal region is examined next and it is important to observe and palpate any sores around the sphincter. During the subsequent rectal exploration, the size and consistency of the prostate glands are ascertained, as well as any increased consistency of the seminal vesicles. In sampling the rectum for gonococci, the mucous membrane just inside the sphincter is swabbed or a probe can be inserted and, after scraping this against the mucosal lining, the sample can be transferred to a swab.

Oral cavity The examination of the anogenital region is followed by an examination of the oral cavity to determine whether papules are present. The tongue is examined closely on the surface, sides and underneath. Culture from the tonsils for gonococci should be included in the culture procedure.

Other examinations The occipital and neck nodes are palpated and the scalp is investigated for the presence of alopecia and infestations. The lymph nodes in the axilla and the skin of the trunk are checked for exanthema. The extremities, including the nodes of the elbow, are also examined. The examination concludes with inspecting the palms and soles to determine whether syphilitic papules are present. The sides of the fingers and the knuckles of the hands are checked for scabies.

After this physical examination, blood samples are taken for the serologic tests for syphilis.

Examination of Women

With the patient in the supine position, the inguinal nodes are palpated and the pubic hair is examined. Secretion samples and cultures for gonococci and *Chlamydia* are taken from the urethra and the genital mucosal membranes are examined for sores and condylomas. If there is secretion, its consistency, odor and color should be noted. After insertion of specula, the vagina and cervix are checked for ulcerations and the cervix is dried with a tampon. Secretion samples for microscopic examination and culture of gonococci are taken from the cervical canal. Secretion samples for detection of *Trichomonas* are taken from the posterior fornix. Finally, the anal region is inspected and samples of secretions are taken from just inside the anal sphincter for gonococcal culture. The examination concludes with vaginal exploration to palpate any pelvic involvement. The rest of the examination is the same as for men.

Ban on intercourse If examination indicates the presence of venereal disease, the patient should avoid intercourse until the disease is no longer contagious. The patient is asked about the source of his/her disease and any subsequent sexual partners. If there is suspicion of venereal disease but the diagnosis is not proved, the patient may be advised to avoid intercourse and be given an explanation of why this is important.

Check-up After the appropriate treatment, the patient is given an appointment for follow-up to ascertain that treatment has been effective. When the check-up shows the patient to be cured, it is important to inform the patient that he/she is no longer contagious and that the disease will not recur unless reinfection occurs.

Gonorrhea

Gonococci

Gonorrhea is caused by a gram-negative diplococcus, the gonococcus *Neisseria gonorrhoeae*. Gonococci can be differentiated from other *Neisseria* types only by biochemical reactions, not by their morphology alone. The gonococci are divided into 5 types according to the morphologic features of the culture.

Experimental infection

Experimental infection of humans has been possible only with cultures of the type I gonococcus. Subsequent culture has shown type I gonococci to be capable of multiplication in the male urethra. Nevertheless, experimental inoculation does not produce symptoms; this, in conjunction with the unsuccessful inoculation attempts using the other types of gonococci, shows that factors other than simply the presence of bacteria are important in causing clinical disease. This is in contrast to the significant clinical risk of infection, which is 85% after coitus with an infected partner. Chimpanzees can be infected with gonococci and transmit the infection by sexual contact. Other animals have not been infected experimentally.

Immunity

Since experimental animals have been used in research, interest in producing vaccines has grown, regardless of the fact that gonorrheal infection normally does not result in immunity after treatment. This does not exclude the possibility that gonorrhea can heal spontaneously, just like other infectious diseases.

Incubation time

Incubation time varies considerably; although normally it is 3–7 days, at times it may be longer. These variations presumably depend on the number of microorganisms inoculated and on the infected person's resistance to disease.

Asymptomatic gonorrhea

Recent years have seen an increase in cases of symptomless or weakly symptomatic infections that are diagnosed only after culture examination. It is difficult to determine whether this increased frequency is relative or absolute. Possible explanations for the former hypothesis can be the increased use of cultures in diagnosis, more intensive tracing of contacts and also routine examination of groups of people, such as those performed in gynecology departments.

Gonorrhea in Men

Symptomatic gonorrhea in men is manifest in only 70% of the infected individuals. Typically it is evidenced by secretions ("dripping") and by frequent and often painful urination. The secretion is generally yellow and thick. It can be so abundant that it actually drips, leaving stiff spots on the underpants—an appearance that gives a clue to the diagnosis. Clinical examination reveals redness and swelling of the urethral meatus. Sometimes the urethritis causes bleeding.

Duration of symptoms

The typical course of the disease is associated with such noticeable and disturbing symptoms that the patient quickly seeks assistance. The secretion is most profuse during the 1st week, decreases thereafter and, after several weeks, can be reduced to a single drop of pus in the morning or a slight pale secretion.

Weakly symptomatic infections

In about 30% of the patients, the secretion can be slight or absent from the beginning. In such cases, the diagnosis is established only by routine examination, such as in the process of tracing the contacts.

Incorrect diagnosis (cystitis) Gonorrhea in men can be misdiagnosed as cystitis. In young men, cystitis is extremely rare. Dysuria, therefore, should not be treated before obtaining a culture for gonococci.

If treatment is easily available and efficacious, complications are rare. Untreated, the infection can spread—most often to the epididymis, less often to the prostate and almost never to the testes.

Epididymitis Epididymitis is extremely painful. It is usually unilateral (mostly on the left side) and accompanied by moderate fever. The most difficult differential diagnosis is testicular torsion, which is afebrile but otherwise has a similar symptomatology and requires immediate surgical intervention.

Prostatitis Prostatitis is an even less frequent complication, which is surprising in view of the anatomical relationship. The patient complains of pressure in the perineum. Rectal examination reveals the prostate to be tender, stretched and enlarged, but smooth. It is seldom that gonorrhea is the cause of an enlarged prostate.

Proctitis In homosexuals the primary site of infection is most often the rectum, but proctitis is seldom symptomatic.

Gonorrhea in Women

Less than half of the women with gonorrhea develop perceptible symptoms. As a result, they tend to have their infection for a longer time before treatment is begun and thus have a greater risk of complications. Infected women comprise a further reservoir of epidemiologic significance. Diagnosis in women is often determined as a result of their being identified as contacts.

Fluor vaginalis; cervicitis When symptoms appear, they tend to be less marked in women than in men. Women who habitually have secretions—e.g., because of trichomoniasis or trachoma inclusion conjunctivitis (TRIC) infection—can ignore a slight change in the quantity or nature of a secretion that is actually due to acute cervicitis. More than half of the women with gonorrhea also have infection with *Trichomonas vaginalis,* which may be the reason for the secretion. A concomitant *Chlamydia* infection can manifest itself by easily traumatized erosions.

Urethritis In infected women, gonococci are found more often in the cervix (90% of the cases) than in the urethra (70%). Urethritis is rarer than cervicitis, but is more often accompanied by symptoms of frequent dysuria, which in itself can cause the patient to visit a physician.

Salpingitis Canalicular spread can cause salpingitis, the most common complication. Often unilateral (as is epididymitis in men), it generally manifests itself in pain and tenderness over the ligaments. Sometimes it is accompanied by fever, especially in conjunction with menstruation. Right-sided salpingitis is difficult to differentiate from appendicitis. Chronic gonorrheic endometritis, salpingitis and salpingo-oophoritis have the same symptoms as infections with other organisms. In less severe cases, the infection produces abdominal pain and irregular menstruations. If salpingitis is bilateral, sterility can result. After effective chemotherapy was instituted in the 1930s, later supplemented with antibiotics, complications were reduced considerably.

Bartholinitis Cultures from the entrance to Bartholin's glands on the medial surface of the labia minora are often positive for gonorrhea. Clinical bartholinitis, however, is rare, although it can occur, associated with pain and swelling and, possibly, with an abscess as well.

Proctitis In about 30% of women with gonorrhea, gonococci can be cultured from the rectum, but proctitis with clinical symptoms is rare. In about 5% of cases, gonococci are found only in the rectum. This infection is generally due to rectal coitus.

Extragenital Gonorrhea

Tonsil gonorrhea Gonococci can be found in the throat of both men and women. This infection is usually symptomless or with only minimal symptoms, but has appeared increasingly in recent years. It is unknown whether there is actually an increased incidence due to changed sexual practices in the form of genito-oral contact. Previously, it was not as common to do throat cultures in search of gonococci. Any diplococci thus found can be misinterpreted as other types of *Neisseria,* especially meningococci.

Dermatitis-arthritis syndrome Hematogenous spread in the form of gonorrheic dermatitis-arthritis syndrome is encountered in both sexes, but most often in women. Symptoms develop in a few days, in women especially in the first 8 days of the menstrual cycle and begin with malaise, slight fever (38–38.5C), migratory arthralgia, especially in the small joints, and finally, a pathognomonic skin eruption. This is localized to the hands (Fig. 4) and feet (Fig. 5) and consists of a few lesions, usually less than 10 in all. These develop within a day and begin as papules less than 5 mm in size, surrounded by a red halo. The following day they become necrotic pustules and may be black because of bleeding. Gonococci can rarely be cultured from the pustules, but are sometimes seen by fluorescent microscopy of a biopsy, which gives a picture of allergic vasculitis.

Arthritis is transitory and sterile. Skin eruptions are so characteristic that they ought to call for immediate examination for gonorrhea. It is usually possible to find gonococci in the throat or the anogenital region. Even if the diagnosis is made on the basis of the clinical picture, it must be verified by demonstration of gonococci in the oroanogenital region.

In patients with this clinical picture, throat gonorrhea seems to be frequent. Partners of the patient with the gonorrheic dermatitis-arthritis syndrome have an increased incidence of this syndrome and an increased incidence of asymptomatic gonorrhea. This suggests that a special type of gonococci are responsible for this course of the disease.

Gonorrheic monarthritis

Untreated gonorrhea can, in rare instances, lead to another type of joint disease, called gonorrheic monarthritis, which most often affects the large joints. These become painful and swollen, containing a considerable amount of exudate from which gonococci can be cultured.

The etiologic diagnosis of the above-mentioned types of gonorrheic arthritis is based solely on the identification of gonococci in the anogenital region, throat or in aspirated joint fluid.

Ophthalmoblenorrhea

Administration of 0.67% silver nitrate eye drops at birth successfully abolishes gonorrheic opthalmoblenorrhea, previously the cause of blindness in many of the children infected with gonorrhea during birth. Gonorrheic conjunctivitis, extremely rare in adults, manifests itself in intense redness and purulent secretion. In both newborns and adults, conjunctivitis is more commonly a complication of urethritis caused by TRIC agents than a result of gonorrheic urethritis.

Vulvo-vaginitis Vulvovaginitis in children was previously attributed to inadequate hygiene. If a genital infection in a child proves to be gonococcal, the sexual organ must be examined.

Diagnosis

Sampling Diagnosis is based on microscopic and culture study. Secretion sample for direct microscopic examination is taken from the urethra in men and from the urethra and cervix in women. Traditionally, a flat or hollowed out urethral probe is used (Fig. 1); any instrument that does not damage the urethral mucous membrane can be used, such as a platinum loop or, for lack of anything better, a common cotton swab. A flat urethral probe is inserted about 0.5–1 cm sagitally; it is rotated and then withdrawn, with the distal part of the probe lying along the floor of the navicular fossa.

In women, the sample is taken from the urethra in a similar way and, after insertion of specula, also from the cervix.

Direct microscopic examination of samples from the rectum or the tonsils is useless because of the abundance of various bacterias in these areas.

The smear is spread on a dry glass slide; it is air-dried and perhaps flame-fixed and then stained.

Staining the preparation 1. For the general physician we recommend the method using a 1% methylene blue solution. The solution is poured on the slide, which is rinsed off immediately and dried with filter paper. This requires only 1 bottle, can be performed in 1 minute and gives the same yield as the Gram stain.

2. Venereal disease clinics doing many examinations use 0.1% methylene blue, kept in special containers, into which the slide is placed for a minimum of 30–60 seconds. With longer times there is no danger of overstaining. The slide is rinsed in ample running water until no more color comes off and is then dried.

In the event that many preparations are being treated at the same time, it is essential to mark the individual slides.

3. Gram's staining method, which stains gonococci red (gram-negative), requires expertise in evaluating the result and much help. It is not recommended for physicians who perform microscopic examination rarely and who do not have experienced technical help. This test does not give a greater number of positive results than the other method, but serves to verify that the intracellular diplococci are gram-negative.

4. Fluorescence microscopy reveals gonococci after addition of fluorescein-marked antigonococcic rabbit serum. The method is still a research procedure.

Microscopic examination

An oil immersion lens is used in the examination and the stained gonococci appear clustered side by side like coffee beans, partly intracellularly in polymorphonuclear leukocytes and partly extracellularly. The intracellular localization is characteristic of gonococci (and meningococci) and, therefore, diagnostic.

Often there are few bacteria, which recommends a careful examination. In men, other types of bacteria are seldom found, but the microscopic diagnosis of women is made more difficult by the presence of many different kinds of microorganisms.

Culture

The smear specimen may be cultured on special mediums. In order to obtain reliable cultures, the time necessary to send the culture to a special laboratory must be kept to a minimum and special mediums (e.g. Thayer-Martin or Stuart) have to be used for transporting it.

In microscopically verified gonorrhea in men, culturing is sometimes indicated to determine resistance to antibodies and also to check on treatment failures. Negative cultures are required traditionally, before a male patient is declared cured. This custom originated at a time when treatment was less reliable than today.

Ideally, if the situation warrants, the follow-up culture can be omitted; e.g., when the patient is asymptomatic or if a test for resistance was done at the first examination and the treatment has been adequate in accordance.

In women, the microscopic diagnosis is so uncertain that a culture should be done. Specimens should routinely be taken from the urethra, the cervical canal, the rectum and possibly from the tonsils. Culture samples taken from the vagina instead of the cervix are reasonably reliable and can be obtained without a speculum; this may be useful when the examination must be done by lay personnel, such as in developing countries.

Rectal and tonsil gonorrhea can be diagnosed only by culture.

Inoculation The specimen is taken using a sterile charcoal-saturated cotton swab. The charcoal increases the surface area of the swab and counteracts the toxic substances in the cotton, which may be bactericidal. The swab is gently scraped against the mucous membrane after secretion has been sampled for direct microscopy. It is important that the rectal sample be taken from the rectal mucous membrane just inside the sphincter and *not* from feces; sampling requires only that the swab be inserted into the anal ring. Use of a urethral scoop or secretion probe has been recommended by some for sample collection, after which the secretion is transferred to a charcoal swab. Specimens are taken from the throat just as for a normal culture from the tonsils, but using a charcoal cotton swab.

The swabs are put directly into a transport medium.

NOTE: Examination for *Chlamydia* should be made before swabbing for gonococci because charcoal interferes with *Chlamydia* cultures.

Transport substrate This substrate contains no nutrients, but keeps the culture moist in a high carbon dioxide and low oxygen atmosphere. In the transport medium, the bacteria will survive, but not grow.

Stuart's medium is clear and opalescent and it contains an indicator that turns blue if the oxygen content is too high. In the event that more than ⅓ of the top of the glass is blue, the specimen must be discarded. The transport tubes should be kept at 4 C and replaced regularly.

Because Stuart's medium contains no nutrients, the transport time must not exceed 24 hours, especially in the summer. To ensure that a negative result is not due to the sampling method or to death of bacteria during transport, tests that gave negative results should be repeated.

Culture medium Culturing of gonococci is done using special mediums that, among other things, contain horse blood, so-called chocolate agar. After several days' growth, the gonococci appear as small, porcelain-like colonies. The selective substrate hinders the growth of strongly penicillin-sensitive gonococci, which must be taken into account when interpreting the results.

Determination of resistance Sensitivity tests can be performed. A disk method is used, in which the individual disks are saturated with antibiotics or sulfonamides. The isolated gonococci's sensitivity to penicillin, tetracyclin, streptomycin and sulfonamides is determined.

Certain gonococci may be lost during transport, and a negative culture does not necessarily disprove a definite microscopic diagnosis. If two consecutive cultures have been done without treatment in between and only the result of one is positive, therapy should be instituted.

Treatment

The extremely effective means of treatment have apparently not had any effect on the frequency of the disease.

Treatment has changed, thanks to pharmacologic developments and in consideration of the constantly changing resistance pattern of the gonococci families. Penicillin is the main means of treating patients who are not allergic to it. The dose, however, has had to be steadily increased during the past 15 years. The treatment aims at quickly establishing a high serum concentration of penicillin, which is then maintained for at least 8–12 hours.

Parenteral therapy

The 2 most important protocols are described below.

1. Benzyl penicillin sodium, 5 million I.U., is dissolved in 8 ml of 0.5 % lidocaine (since penicillin dissolves hypotonically) and given intramuscularly in the gluteal region. Half an hour before injection, 1 gm of probenecid is given orally to prevent renal tubular elimination of the penicillin. This treatment procedure has been used with success wherever gonococcal strains with reduced sensitivity occur very frequently; therefore, it can be chosen with confidence if a determination of resistance is not available or cannot be made.

2. In areas where most of the gonococcal types are strongly sensitive to penicillin, treatment with benzyl penicillin sodium, 1 million I.U., plus procain penicillin, 1.2 million I.U., given simultaneously, intramuscularly, has proved to be especially effective. This treatment is preferred in Sweden, for example. Other schematic penicillin dosages for parenteral use cannot be recommended at present.

Oral therapy

Oral treatment is easy, painless and reduces the chances of life-threatening anaphylactic shock. In the event that taking the pills cannot be supervised at the place of treatment, the patient must have the desire and ability to cooperate and must understand the importance of following the instructions given by the physician.

1. Most oral penicillin preparations give too low serum concentrations and, furthermore, concentrations vary considerably among individuals. In uncomplicated gonorrhea, ampicillin 3.5 g orally given with probenicid is usually effective. If probenicid is not available, the dose of ampicillin can be divided into two equal doses taken five hours apart. Amoxicillin (3 g orally) plus 1 gram probenecid gives as good a result as ampicillin.

2. Tetracycline is also effective against gonorrhea and can be used if a penicillin allergy is suspected. Dosage could be, for example, tetracycline 500 mg orally, then 500 mg qid for four days.

3. Erythromycin is also effective when given in a dose of 500 mg orally/qid for five days. This treatment should be preferred to tetracycline for pregnant women.

4. Chemotherapy with sulfonamides was recommended exclusively from 1939 to 1944 and has had a revival with the combination preparation sulfamethoxazole with trimethoprim and Bactrim, which is given in 2 doses of 5 tablets each, 8 hours apart. This treatment can lose its effectiveness, however, if the bacteria are sulfonamide-resistant. Treatment is indicated above all when the sore on the genitals is not definitely known not to be of syphilitic origin—in other words, if the spirochete examination was negative.

Complications If complications occur, treatment with penicillin or tetracycline should be continued for 6–10 days. If treatment was started with penicillin G procaine, this should be given once followed by ampicillin 500 mg orally qid. If ampicillin plus probenicid was given as an initial dose, the treatment should be continued with ampicillin 500 mg orally for ten days. Similarly tetracycline treatment should be continued for ten days, erythromycin for 5–10 days.

Hospitalized patients with pelvic inflammatory disease can be treated with crystalline penicillin G 20 million units IV daily until improvement. Patients with gonococcal dermatitisarthritis syndrome may also benefit from an initial three-day treatment with 10 million units IV for at least three days with crystalline penicillin G, but oral treatment with ampicillin is equally effective. It should be started with 3.5 grams orally and probenicid 1 gram orally followed by ampicillin 500 mg orally qid for at least seven days.

Masked syphilis With the introduction of penicillin therapy, concern was raised that the moderate dosage (i.e., 300,000 I.U. of procain penicillin) would mask simultaneously contracted syphilis, which consequently could only be recognized after the disease has caused irreparable damage. Experience has not supported this concern since, on the contrary, tertiary and latent stages of syphilis have become rare. Although penicillin treatment given for gonorrhea seems to cure rather than to mask a simultaneously contracted syphilis, this does not necessarily apply when the syphilis infection was acquired *before* the gonorrheic infection and when treatment for gonorrhea is given late in the syphilis incubation period.

Resistance of gonococci to antibiotics When sulfonamides were introduced, nearly all gonococci were sensitive. Ten years later, more than half of the strains exhibited resistance to sulfonamides. Similar resistance is not exhibited to penicillin, although the number of strains showing reduced sensitivity to penicillin has increased periodically. At present, the number of strains with decreased sensitivity to penicillin is declining. Gonococcal strains may be classified according to their sensitivity to penicillin into 2 groups. The distribution of resistance shows large geographic variations, which may be the result of therapeutic traditions.

Gonococcal strains with greatly reduced sensitivity are found predominantly in areas where penicillin treatment is given in insufficient doses—for example, as a consequence of self-medication. This applies especially to East Asia, where antibiotics have been bought and sold on the black market. These chromosomal mutants can be eradicated by increasing the dosage of penicillin.

Penicillin resistent strains produce beta lactamate or penicillinase and were first observed in 1975 in patients returning from the Far East. These strains have spread within the United States. They are caused by a plasmid or an R-factor. This plasmid is by itself sexually transmissible. The resistent gonococci can be reliably treated only with spectinomycin.

Patients infected with resistent strains of gonococci are still few in number. To prevent speading of the infection it is of special importance to find and treat all contacts.

Resistance pattern Determination of resistance is primarily of interest as a guide to treatment. A gonococcal strain that is isolated after the completion of treatment, in the event of a recurrence because of treatment failure, will show the same resistance pattern as the originally isolated gonococci. If the resistance pattern differs considerably from the original one, it probably indicates reinfection.

The resistance pattern is also of interest in contact tracing, since the relevant contact will have the same resistance pattern.

Ban on intercourse Intercourse is forbidden when the diagnosis of gonorrhea has been established and the interdiction is usually maintained until cure. "Recurrence" as a result of treatment failure will appear within 1 week in men and within 2 weeks in women, and the duration of the ban on intercourse is set correspondingly.

Follow-up Ideally, follow-up includes culture examination and should be completed within 2–3 weeks. Previously, patients were examined for long periods, but the gonococci revealed by the last examinations may well have been new infections.

Prognosis Treatment performed correctly and reasonably early in the course of illness will effect cure in all cases. The disease normally has no sequellae. Sterility after salpingitis occurs in about 2% of patients. Urethral constriction, which usually occurred in men and was considered to be a complication of gonorrhea, was apparently due to the treatment with silver nitrate irrigation, which was the predominant method before antibiotic treatment was introduced.

In view of the popular misconceptions on the unfavorable prognosis of venereal disease, it is important to inform the patient that the disease is wholly curable and benign if the treatment is sufficient.

Serologic follow-up The patient is advised to return 3 months after completion of treatment for a serologic test, to detect possible masked syphilis.

Nongonococcal Urethritis

The incidence of this group of diseases has increased more rapidly than gonorrhea. Non-gonorrheic urethritis is as difficult to treat, and is more often followed by complications than gonorrhea.

Nongonorrheic urethritis can be due to a number of known causes, but in many cases its etiology is unknown.

In venereal disease clinics, the patients who most often present with symptoms are men. In women, some of the similar diseases are cervicitis and portio erosions, but the symptoms of these are often minimal. The seemingly lower frequency in women may be due to the fact that, on the one hand, they have fewer symptoms and, on the other, patients with symptoms more often turn to their physician, because the irritation is not interpreted as a symptom of a sexually transmitted disease.

The incubation time for nongonorrheic urethritis varies from a few days to a month, depending on etiologic factors. The patient's main complaint is usually urethral secretion, but stinging and itching also occur. The symptoms may be present only in the morning, in the form of sticking together of the urethral opening. Often the complaint is only a feeling of increased moistness in the urethra. If secretion occurs, it ranges from pale to purulent. Spots may appear on the underpants. Historically, information on a long incubation time suggests the diagnosis of nongonorrheic urethritis and often there will be history of previous, similar symptoms.

Nongonorrheic urethritis can occur simultaneously with gonorrhea; in that case, secretion continues in spite of adequate antigonorrheal treatment, although it often changes character and becomes less purulent. It used to be called post-gonococcal discharge.

Chlamydia Trachomatis Infection

The most frequent cause of NGU is infection with *Chlamydia trachomatis*. This was previously called *C. bedsonia* or TRIC agent (trachoma-inclusion conjunctivitis agent). These differ from viruses by having a discreet cell wall and from bacteria by being able to multiply only within the host cells. There are two species of *Chlamydia*, *C. psitaci*, which causes ornithosis, and *C. trachomatis*, of which some serotypes cause lymphogranuloma venereum, some endemic trachoma and others the sexually transmitted conditions described below.

Symptoms in men

C. trachomatis can be isolated in about 40–50% of all men with non-gonorrhoic urethritis (NGU), whereas *Chlamydia* is rarely found in the urethra in controls without urethritis. The incubation time is 4–30 days, usually 7–21 days. Simultaneous infection with *Chlamydia* and gonococci is common, and since *Chlamydia* are unaffected by penicillin treatment, the clinical result will often be a cured gonorrhoea followed by a post-gonococcal *Chlamydia* urethretitis.

Complications

If untreated, the infection may spread to the epididymis. In younger men *Chlamydia* are the most common cause of epididymitis, while in men over 35 soliform bacteria are the usual causes. In chronic prostatitis *Chlamydia* occur in mixed infections with *Trichomonas vaginalis*, herpes virus, and gonococci.

Symptoms in women

Between 20 and 40% of women attending a VD clinic will harbor *Chlamydia* in the cervix, less often in the urethra and the rectum. A positive finding is common in contacts with men having NGU.

**Compli-
cations**

In the last few years a number of studies have convincingly shown *Chlamydia* to be a common cause of genital disease in women. *Chlamydia* are very often demonstrated in cervical erosions which easily bleed at a touch with a speculum. Whether *Chlamydia* cause the erosions is uncertain, possibly erosions are easily infected. Acute salpingitis is caused by *Chlamydia* in one-third of the cases, *Chlamydia* being recovered from the tubae by laparoscopy. The role of *Chlamydia* in chronic cervical infection dyspareunia and sterility is not clear.

Recovery of *Chlamydia* in non-venerological materials is low, but symptomless genital infections have been established in females who have been examined because of *Chlamydia* conjunctitis.

**Extra-
genital
infections**

In adults of both sexes *Chlamydia* may cause inclusion conjunctivitis. Swimming-pool conjunctivitis has been ascribed to infection with genital strains of *Chlamydia trachomatis*. In many cases *Chlamydia* can be recovered from the rectum, but symptoms of proctitis are rare. *Chlamydia* have sometimes been recovered from the pharynx, but symptoms of sore throat are uncommon.

**The
newborn**

During birth the *Chlamydia* infection may be transmitted to the infant giving rise to inclusion conjunctivitis. This mucopurulent conjunctivitis appears in some newborn infants and may have late effects after neovascularization in the cornea and scar-forming conjunctivitis.

The infection may spread to the nose, pharynx and trachea and may cause a pneumonia with spotwise infiltrates. Tachypnea, coughing and cyanosis are the prevailing symptoms.

Diagnosis Facilities for routine culture of *Chlamydia* are rarely available. Suitable culture media are hens' eggs and McCoy's cell cultures. A methylene blue stained smear from the male urethra often shows abundant polymorphonuclear leukocytes and large blast-like cells with a large darkly stained nucleus and a diameter twice that of the polymorphonuclears.

If gonococci are present together with the blast-like cells, the patient is likely to develop a postgonococcal urethritis. When treated with penicillin and if facilities for Giemsa staining are available, the preparation may show inclusions as a sign of *Chlamydia* infection.

A microimmunofluorescence test seems to be the diagnostic method of the future, since it is positive in almost everyone with *Chlamydia* urethritis and rarely in controls.

Treatment The preferred treatment of *Chlamydia* infections is tetracyline given in full systemic doses for at least two weeks, but some treat for a longer period. Erythromycin is equally effective and so is sulfamethoxazol.

It is of importance also to treat the sexual partner at the same time even if they are without symptoms. This must be done in order to avoid reinfections from the same source., and to prevent a female partner from developing serious complications later on. If the female partner is pregnant, avoid tetracycline.

Ureaplasma (Mycoplasma)

These organisms are commonly found in the urogenital region of promiscuous patients. *Ureaplasma hominis* is presumably an incidental finding without pathologic significance. *Ureaplasma urealyticum (T. mycoplasma)* may possibly be pathogenic but only if found in large numbers. Experimental autoinnoculation has been shown to cause urethritis, fever and arthralgia.

Ureaplasma urealyticum disappears within one

week's treatment with tetracycline, to which they are highly sensitive.

Bacterial NGU and Allied Genital Infections

E. coli and *Staphylococcus aureus* can cause bacterial urethritis. The finding of coli in the urethra must be regarded as pathological, whereas *Staphylococci* can be saprophytes. A culture showing *Staphylococcus albus* may be ignored.

Many other types of neisseriae than gonococci may be present in the urethra. Among them mimea can cause urethritis. They are diplococci resembling gonococci on microscopy, but they can be distinguished by fermentation. Mimeae are considerably less sensitive to penicillin than gonococci.

Streptococci Group B

Streptococci of group B have been isolated in VD clinics more often than in controls. Thus, one-third of all women with gonorrhoea simultaneously harbored group B Streptococci, whereas this was only the case for one sixth of the males with gonorrhoea. It seems that group B streptococci give rise to a vaginitis with pain, erythema and discharge. Group B streptococci have also been isolated from the urethra of males with NGU, but they rarely cause symptoms. It is possible to treat infections with group B *Streptococci* with ampicillin. Infections with group B *Streptococci* are of special importance in pregnant women, because they can cause lethal septicemia in newborn who are infected during birth. A case rate of 3/1000 deliveries is estimated.

Hemophilus vaginalis

Hemophilus vaginalis has a low degree of pathogenicity and virulence but can cause a frothy vaginal discharge with a foul smell.

Characteristic microscopic findings are few leukocytes and large numbers of epithelial cell which are filled with Gram-negative rods. These cells are diagnostic. Male consorts rarely have symptoms but should be treated at the same time as their contacts, ampicillin or tetracyline are both effective.

Herpes genitalis (see p. 38).
Candida urethritis (see p. 36).
Trichomonas urethritis (see p. 35).

Treatment

It is not possible to give a standard treatment procedure for an infection with numerous causes. Since the infection is sexually transmitted, however, it is extremely important for any treatment to be given, not only to the patient, but also to the patient's partner(s). The explanation for the frequently observed recurrences is probably that simultaneous treatment of the partner(s) has been neglected.

If no gonococci are found in the smear from a man with urethritis an examination for *trichomonas, Candida albicans* and a culture for other bacteria should be performed. *Trichomonas* urethritis should be treated with metronidazole and bacterial non-gonorrheic urethritis with antibiotics in accordance with the sensitivity pattern.

If the etiological factors have not been determined *C. trachomatis*, or rarely *Ureaplasma urealyticum*, are likely causes of the urethritis. The patient should be treated with tetracycline one gram daily for at least two weeks. It is important to continue treatment even if the symptoms disappear rather quickly after commencement of the treatment. Sexual partners should be examined for gonorrhea and treated as above, i.e., a full course of tetracycline for at least two weeks. Treatment failures are commonly traced to reinfection or treatment for an insufficiently long period of time.

Reiter's Syndrome

Reiter's Syndrome may start with enteritis or with urethritis, and occurs preferably in patients with HLA-B 27 (80%) and almost exclusively in younger men. The rarity in women is unexplained.

Trachomata (group B) When the syndrome starts with urethritis, *Chlamydia* are often involved, but sometimes gonococci are also found. Their eradication has no influence on the course of illness. It is unknown whether the *Chlamydia* actually trigger the development of symptoms in persons with a particular genetic constitution.

Symptoms Joint symptoms develop days or weeks after the urethritis. The first affected are the sacroiliac, and other joints soon become involved. Inflammation in the plantar fascia is characteristic, and in the acute stage, pain on walking is seen. The temperature is slightly elevated, there may be conjunctivitis and anterior iritis.

The mucous membranes may be involved, in the form of a circinate balanitis or vulvitis, and scaly, psoriasiform papules may appear on the palms and soles. This manifestation is called keratodermia blenorrhagica. The acute phase lasts from 1–3 months, but there is a high risk of recurrence. Ankylosing arthritis is late sequel. Traction from the shrinkage process in the plantar fascia can be shown by x-ray in the form of the heel spur, which in itself can give secondary pain on walking.

Laboratory investigations reveal a greatly increased sedimentation rate, and serumelectrophoresis shows a considerable increase in α-2-globulins. A positive lygranum complement fixation reaction is often found with Reiter's syndrome, and aspiration from the joints involved have shown *Chlamydia* or *Mycoplasma*.

Trichomoniasis

Trichomoniasis is the most frequent sexually transmitted disease. In females, it causes vaginitis, cervicitis and cystitis, whereas in men, it most often causes urethritis. *Trichomonas vaginalis* occurs only in the genital tract, unlike other *trichomonas* species, which are found in the intestines and oral cavity.

Trichomonas vaginalis is 15–30 µ long, twice the size of polymorpho-nuclear leukocytes, pear-shaped, and has 4 flagella in the wide end and an undulating membrane along one side.

Epidemiology Trichomonas vaginalis infections are especially common among women who are seen in VD clinic, and are found in the majority of women with gonorrhea.

Gynecological patients show a frequency of about 5%. In male consorts to women with *Trichomonas vaginalis*, infection can be established in more than 30% in the first weeks after intercourse, but with a rapid decline due to spontaneous cures. The infection is promoted by repeated contact, and by damage of the mucous membrane by a simultaneous gonorrhea.

In women the infection can be transmitted indirectly, for example from toilet seats, since the organisms can survive in a moist atmosphere at room temperature.

Many infections are asymptomatic, and men usually have slight symptoms.

Clinical features The incubation time is up to four weeks, and usually symptoms are most pronounced immediately after menstruation. The major symptoms in women are abundant grey, white or yellow and frothy vaginal mucosa. The maceration, redness and stinging may extend to the vulva and the genitofemoral areas. Pronounced itching suggests an infection with *Candida albicans* rather than with *T. vaginalis*.

In both sexes *Trichomonas* may cause urethritis and cystitis. Hematuria may result from trigonum cystitis. In men, prostatitis can be diagnosed by microscopical or cultural examination of prostatic secretion or of an ejaculate. Hematospermia may result from a trichomonal epididymitis. Occasionally a minimal balanopostitis is found.

Diagnosis Smears in women are taken from the vagina, where the posterior fornix gives the highest yield; in men smears are taken from the urethra. Prostatic secretions may also be examined, as well as a urinary sediment.

Trichomonas vaginalis can be detected microscopically by mixing a drop secretion with physiologic saline solution on a glass slide, and covering with a cover slip. A phase-contrast or dark-field microscope is particularly helpful. *Trichomonas* can be stained with Papanicolau stain, and will be revealed in a vaginal-cytological examination. The most reliable methods of detection is culture after forwarding the specimen in a transport medium.

Treatment Treatment consists of chemotherapy with metronidazol (Flagyl). The dosage for metronidazol is 200 mg three times daily for 7 days or 2 g in a single dose. This occasionally causes headaches, furry tongue and exanthema. Alcohol intolerance may be experienced during treatment.

Detection of trichomonas vaginalis should lead to treating the patient's partner(s) in order to prevent reinfection from contacts. The first consideration should be the possibility of reinfection from an unreported and therefore non-treated contact. It is advisable to give the patient enough medications for three courses of treatment.

Candidiasis

Candida albicans, or thrush, is a yeast that may be an incidental finding, for example, from gonococci culture; under certain circumstances, however, it can produce a symptomatic infection. It is essential to distinguish the difference between asymptomatic *Candida* colonization and clinical infection.

The disease is detected with increasing frequency. Growth of the fungus can be promoted by changes in the bacterial flora or hormone balance. In younger women *Candida* infections occur especially during the use of oral contraceptives or pregnancy. In older persons, it may be a complication of diabetes, and in all age groups it occurs after prolonged treatment with antibiotics or cytostatic drugs.

In young persons the infection is usually sexually transmitted. This always applies to men with *Candida* urethritis, since *Candida* is never found in the urethra in hematogenous candidiasis.

Detection can be achieved by direct microscopic examination or KOH-treatment of a smear or by a culture study using Nickerson's medium, in which brown colonies grow to a recognizable size within very few days.

Clinical presentation

Candida can be detected in about 5 % of all gynecologic patients, but only a third will be symptomatic. In women, the chief complaint is an intense itching in the genital region; simultaneously there may be a cheesy, white secretion. The mucous membranes are covered with a whitish film or a more massive cheesy coating, but erosions occur as well.

In younger women, *Candida* infections occur especially in connection with use of contraceptives or with pregnancy.

Ten percent of men with *Candida*-infected partners develop balanitis, which can be intermittent and has small papules that can erode. Urethritis may occur. Men may have itching on the glans and prepuce from *Candida* and sometimes this is the only complaint; this pruritus is especially noticeable after coitus.

Treatment Treatment is given only to symptomatic patients and is topical. It consists of nystatin (mycostatin), Natamycin (Pimafucin) or amphotericin B (Fungilin), which is specifically effective against *Candida*. In women, the medication is given as vaginal suppositories; in men, it is dispensed as a cream which is to be used for 2 weeks. For urethritis, the urethra can be rinsed with dilute mycostatin suspension. It is advisable to treat the patient's contact to prevent reinfection. In recurrence in women, reinfection from the gastrointestinal tract must be considered; a renewed therapy should be supplemented with oral mycostatin tablets (2 given 3 times daily for 14 days). Mycostatin is minimally absorbed from the gastrointestinal tract. (Note: griseofulvin is not effective against yeast infections.)

Broad-spectrum antimycotics can be used in the treatment, such as Miconazole, oxyquinolones, and Triphenylmethane dyes (methylrosaniline chloride).

Herpes Progenitalis

Herpes progenitalis is the most common cause of recurring genital ulcerations. Eighty percent of cases are due to infection with *Herpesvirus hominis* type II, a DNA virus closely related to, but not identical with, herpesvirus type I, which causes herpes labialis. The incubation time is unknown, but the occurrence, attributable to intimate contact, takes place within the 1st week after intercourse. The virus is latent in the regional neural ganglia. The disease can recur by various provocations such as lowered resistance due to fever or menstruation and after increased sexual activity. Herpes can be cultured more often than expected from men with gonorrhea, and possibly gonorrhea can activate a latent herpes infection.

Clinical presentation

Eruption begins with an itching erythema that develops into closely set small vesicles within 24 hours, sometimes in a cloverleaf pattern. Within a few days, the vesicles break, leaving small ulcerations that can coalesce, forming one large ulcer, that can be secondarily infected. Scar formation is absent or minimal. The regional nodes are slightly swollen and tender.

In men, eruption occurs on the skin of the penis, prepuce or glans (Fig. 11), but sometimes in the pubic area. Herpes virus also causes urethritis, commonly together with eruption on the skin. The major symptom is violent pain at micturation. Urethroscopy occasionally reveals erosions. Microscopy of urethral smears stained with methlene blue or Giemsa stain show multinucleated giant cells.

Herpes type II infections can be located on the mucous membrane in women, but also in the genitofemoral area, on the hips and buttocks. Both the ulcerations and the regional nodes are often more painful in women than in men; in particular, the primary ulcerations in the vulva can be so painful that bed rest and application of compresses are necessary. Tender inguinal nodes may be the initial symptom and sometimes the dominant complaint.

Herpetic ulcerations on the cervix are underdiagnosed. They are seen as "erosions," whereas the tender regional glands manifest themselves in dyspareunia and pain in the pelvis or over the ligaments, especially at menstruation. Dysuria and secretion can be the chief complaints.

Neonatal infections
Herpes virus II has caused generalized herpes infections in newborns infected during birth. The risk of neonatal infection is 10% if the infection occurs after the 32nd week of gestation, and 40% if the mother has herpes genitalis at the time of birth.

One third of the children have benign localized herpes eruption, while the remainder have generalized infection, which is often lethal. Cerebrospinal damage develops in those who survive. Because of the serious consequences for the newborn, pregnant women with frequently recurring herpes progenitalis should have a weekly culture for herpes virus in the last months of pregnancy. A herpes eruption at the time of delivery warrants a Caesarean section.

There is suggestive evidence that infections with herpes virus II promote the later development of cervical carcinoma.

Diagnosis
Herpes progenitalis, after rupture of the vesicles, can be mistaken for primary syphilis. Closer inspection will often reveal that a larger sore is composed of several smaller, coalescent circular ulcers. If there is doubt about the diagnosis, the patient should be referred for dark-field microscopic examination.

Taking a smear from a herpetic lesion is considerably more painful to the patient than taking a smear from a syphilitic chancre. The indication of pain, however, is not sufficient for making the differential diagnosis.

History of previous lesions with similar localization that healed after 1 or 2 weeks suggests the diagnosis of herpes genitalis. A smear from the base of retained or newly burst vesicles, placed on a glass slide after Giemsa or Wright staining, will reveal large, clear, ballooning virus cells and polymorphonuclear giant cells (Fig. 12).

If facilities are available, the herpes virus can be cultured from the vesicles or, if they are ruptured, from the floor of vesicles within five days of the eruption. Two herpes complement fixation tests made at 14-day intervals will show an increased titer in the case of a primary infection. In about 80 % of the adult population, tests show a weakly positive herpes complement-fixing reaction from previous infection. Complement fixation testing is not routine in the investigation of herpes virus type II.

Treatment Treatment of herpes is not rewarding. 5-iodooxyuridine which inhibits DNA synthesis may shorten the course if the treatment is started early enough and the preparation is given in a sufficient concentration. 5% or 40% iodooxyuridine in dimethylsulphoxide should be applied at least every three hours. Painting with proflavine followed by ultraviolet radiation has been abandoned, because of possible carcogenicity. Human gamma globulin has been utilized.

Wet compresses on the mucous membranes and bland cream on the skin can be used. Local steroid treatment is debatable because of a theoretical risk of virus spreading.

If syphilis has not been ruled out, water should be used for the compress before darkfield investigation is undertaken, since disinfecting or antibacterial substances will kill the spirochetes locally.

Since the disease is contagious, sexual activity should be avoided when ulcerations are present. Condoms should be used during intercourse.

Syphilis

History Syphilis spread in an epidemic in Europe around 1500, presumably brought there in connection with the discovery of America. Syphilis and gonorrhea were considered the same disease until 1839, when Philippe Ricord showed, by inoculation experiments on man, that there actually were 2 diseases. In 1905, Hoffmann and Schaudinn isolated *Spirochaeta pallida* and in 1908 Salvarsan (discovered by Ehrlich) replaced the previous mercury treatment. Since 1945 penicillin has been the preferred treatment. A serologic test for syphilis was first described in 1906 (Wassermann and his colleagues). The natural history of the disease is known from Norwegian research begun by Boeck.

Etiology

Spiro- *Spirochaeta pallida,* or *Treponema pallidum,* is a 5–
chaeta 20-µm long spiral with 6–20 regular turns, which has
pallida characteristic movements, both around the longitudinal axis and bending from the middle. It differs from nonpathogenic spirochetes both in structure and in movements. The organisms can also be found on the oral and genital mucous membranes. *S. pallida* cannot be cultured on artificial media; therefore, animal passages are required (e.g., rabbit testicles are often used). Mitosis takes around 30 hours, which explains the long incubation of the disease and the necessity for lengthy treatment, in view of the fact that spirochetes are susceptible to antibiotics only during mitosis. Spirochetes survive for only a few hours outside a warm-blooded organism, but are viable in transfusion blood preserved at 4 C for up to 72 hours. Spirochetes die if they dry out, if exposed to even weak antiseptics or warmed to 40 C, which was the basis for fever therapy.

It is not certain whether spirochetes penetrate an intact skin or mucous membrane or whether microscopic abrasions are sufficient for them to produce infection. In either case, why is the primary lesion usually solitary?

Clinical Features

The incubation time is 2–4 weeks, but can extend to 3 months. The number of spirochetes inoculated influences the duration of incubation.

Primary ulceration A hard chancre is an ulcer up to 10 mm in diameter, which develops within a few days. It is yellowish-red and the surface is clean or lightly stained by pus. Although the painless induration is considered a major characteristic, it must be stressed that about 25% of the chancres are painful and that the induration is missing in many men and more women.

The chancre is most often localized around the genitalia. In men, it is most frequent on the inside of the prepuce and in the coronal sulcus, especially around the frenulum (Fig. 13). When located on the prepuce, it may cause edema (Fig. 14) and thus phimosis, which makes examination difficult. In women, the common sites are the posterior commissures, labia or circumclitoral area. Chancres in the vagina and on the cervix seldom are symptomatic and the infection often goes unrecognized until the secondary lesions develop. Cervical chancres are sometimes thought to be "erosions".

Days to weeks after the appearance of the chancre, regional lymph nodes become swollen and hard. The swelling is initially unilateral and not tender unless there is a mixed infection. The lymph nodes are freely movable, do not adhere to each other, and never suppurate. When such swelling of the lymph nodes is found together with a genital sore, suspicion of a syphilitic infection must be high. Sometimes the lymph vessel on the dorsal side of the penis or in the clitoris area can be palpated. Cervical chancres are not accompanied by palpable inguinal nodes.

Regional lymphadenopathy may not have developed at the time of the first visit.

Extra-genital chancres Chancres may appear on the lips and tonsils, especially after orogenital contact. Chancres around the anal sphincter and close to it can occur after anal coitus and are found almost exclusively in homosexual men. Anal chancres may appear alone, mimicking fissures.

Untreated, the chancre disappears after 6–8 weeks and may leave a scar.

Secondary syphilis The secondary form is seen only after untreated primary infections. Syphilis becomes generalized 8–12 weeks after infection, which means that the infection begins to spread at a time when the chancres are still present. One fourth of the patients who seek medical treatment for secondary syphilic manifestations have no recollection or signs of primary lesions.

Secondary syphilis is a septicemia involving all organs and causing an initial malaise, headache and slight fever. Generalized lymphadenopathy is a feature producing palpable nodes in the occipital, inguinal and elbow areas. Thereafter, a macular rash develops, consisting of numerous, barely noticeable (up to 10 mm) erythemous lesions, especially along the sides of the trunk and the flexural aspects of extremities. The exanthem is best viewed with oblique lighting. Lesions are not infiltrated and their color disappears by pressing with a glass slide (diascopy). The rash is not itchy and may escape the patient's notice. The exanthem may disappear within a few weeks, but when it continues, the individual lesions become papular, infiltrated and scaly and, to the unpracticed eye, similar to those of pityriasis rosea and guttate psoriasis. A serological test, recommended for these patients, will be positive in secondary lues. In psoriatics the scaling is psoriatic since syphilitic vasculitis provokes a Koebner phenomenon.

In the secondary period, intermittent exacerbations occur, with increasing infiltration and scaliness. Papules on the palms and soles (Figs. 16 and 17) are important, almost pathognomonic findings, but they are often misdiagnosed. In moist areas, especially the mouth (Fig. 20) and the anogenital region, macerated papules may develop 3–4 months after the infection, in other words, 4–6 weeks after the occurrence of exanthem. These papules coalesce and become flat, sharply demarcated lesions with a macerated surface (condylomata lata). They contain myriads of spirochetes. This manifestation ("wet contact") enhances the infectious character of the disease.

The secondary outbreak may be of short duration; in any case, after 2 years, the infection will no longer be symptomatic. The disease then converts to a latent stage. Note, however, that many patients, even without treatment, do not go through all stages. This presumably relates to the individual's immunity.

Latent syphilis The latent phase has no clinical symptoms, but an investigation of the patient's serum will give positive serologic test for syphilis (STS), although with a decreasing frequency in the tests, while spirochete tests are consistently positive. The infection in these patients will only be diagnosed if a routine blood test is performed. The frequency of latent lues decreased sharply in the 1950s, after the introduction of penicillin for acute infectious diseases, which suggests that penicillin, even given in small doses, can be curative if the patient's immune mechanisms are adequate.

Tertiary syphilis Tertiary syphilis is so rare today that it actually deserves mention only in large textbooks. The manifestations are divided into either benign, i.e., skin and bone changes, or malignant, which affect the vessels and central nervous system (CNS). Skin changes result from granulomatous or necrotic gumma. These lesions, often forming a serpiginous pattern, heal after antisyphilitic treatment, but leave scars. Bone lesions are destructive, resulting in secondary joint involvement and saddle nose. The serious tertiary syphilitic vascular symptoms are aortic aneurysms and involvement of the aortic valves, resulting in aortic insufficiency.

The pathology in the CNS may involve the brain, with development of dementia paralytica, or the spinal cord, causing tabes dorsalis.

Tertiary symptoms develop in only one third of untreated patients and do not become manifest earlier than 10–15 years after infection. Symptoms are subsequent to scarring as a result of arteritis; once developed, the vascular and nerve lesions are not improved by treatment, only their progress is arrested.

Congenital syphilis Untreated syphilis in a pregnant woman can be transmitted through the placenta from the 4th month of pregnancy to birth. The infection may result in late abortion or, possibly, stillbirth. If the child is born alive, the infection is generalized from the start. Some of the effects are papular rash, especially in the diaper area, rhinitis and hepatomegaly. The papular lesions in infants are extremely contagious. The child can be asymptomatic at birth, but later develop syphilis congenita tarda. Symptoms of congenital lues that may be noticeable later include labyrinthine deafness, interstitial keratitis and tooth anomalies (Hutchinson's triad).

If ante-natal examinations include a serologic examination for syphilis, after diagnosis, treatment can be instituted and the child can be cured in utero. Congenital syphilis occurs rarely.

Pregnancy may cause a "false positive" nontreponemal STS test. The *Treponema pallidum* immobilization (TPI) and *fluorescent treponemal antibody* (FTA) tests will then be negative.

Treatment for pregnant patients

1. If the pregnant patient has had syphilis before, but the serologic study in the present pregnancy examination is negative, there is no need to repeat treatment.

2. If the treponemal test is positive and the nonlipoidal STS is negative in a patient previously given sufficient treatment, there is no need to repeat treatment.

3. If both nonlipoidal and treponemal tests are positive and the patient has had an adequate treatment, there is no need for re-treatment.

A child born to a mother who is STS-positive may also show positive serum reactions as a result of passively transferred antibodies. The nonlipoidal STS and TPI will show the same titer as the mother's. On the other hand, the antibodies that can be revealed by Meinicke's as well as other flocculation methods cannot pass through an undamaged placenta. The passively transferred antibodies are not an indication for treatment, but the blood test should be repeated after 6 months, at which time passively transferred antibodies will have disappeared. If the mother has had a primary syphilis during the pregnancy, the child should be examined clinically and serologically every 3 months during the 1st year. These apparently overzealous rules stem from traditions of the time of Salvarsan treatment. Their value is not documented.

Microscopic Diagnosis

Dark-field microscopy Samples are taken for microscopy using a urethral probe along the margin of the lesion, which is gently squeezed to obtain tissue fluid. The secretion is mixed with a drop of saline, covered with a coverslip and examined through an oil immersion lens. Traditionally, a dark-field microscope is used, but a phase-contrast microscope is fully acceptable. The microscopic diagnosis requires considerable experience, since it can be difficult to differentiate *S. pallida* from the nonpathogenic spirochetes found as saprophytes on the mucous membrane.

Under the present conditions, syphilis occurs so seldom that only specialists can obtain sufficient practice in the identification. If possible, it is advisable to refer a patient with a suspicious genital lesion to a specialist. Application of water compress for 1 or 2 days facilitates the detection of spirochetes, especially from a secondarily infected lesion. Other treatment should be avoided, since the spirochetes are sensitive to low concentrations of antiseptics and any other antibiotics.

If spirochetes cannot be found in the lesion or they cannot be identified beyond doubt as *S. pallida,* puncturing of the local lymph node may be performed. This is done with a hypodermic needle while the swollen lymph node is held between two fingers. Several drops of saline solution are injected and aspirated. Any spirochetes detected in the aspirate are pathogenic, since nonpathogenic spirochetes do not invade the body.

In contrast to gonococci, *S. pallida* cannot be cultured.

Serologic Diagnosis

Syphilitic infection produces 2 types of antibodies, i.e., antitreponemal and antilipoidal.

Treponemal antibodies Antitreponemal antibodies are specific for an infection with treponemes. Detection is achieved through various modifications of serologic tests that use spirochetes as antigens.

FTA-ABS Most countries use the FTA-ABS (Fluorescent Treponema Antibody ABSorption test), which is extremely sensitive and capable of detecting the disease early in the primary stage. This test uses nonpathogenic spirochetes (Reiter spirochetes), which, in contrast to *S. pallida,* can be cultured on an artificial medium. Antitreponemal antibodies in a patient's serum will be adsorbed to these spirochetes and detected with fluorescein-marked antiglobulin.

TPI Antibodies in the patient's serum can immobilize spirochetes. This property is the basis for the TPI (Treponema Pallidum Immobilization) reaction. TPI uses *S. pallida* (Nichol's strain). These pathogenic spirochetes are cultured in rabbit testicles and survive in a special medium, preserving their mobility for several days. If treatment is begun early during the primary stage, the TPI and FTA-ABS tests do not demonstrate reactivity. If treatment is not instituted early, TPI and FTA-ABS results remain positive. The antitreponemal tests are especially useful as a supplementary examination in patients who have antilipid antibodies but no clinical history of syphilis. If the TPI result is positive in such a case, this indicates that the patient either has or has had syphilis and that treatment is required. If the treponemal STS test is negative and the antilipid test is positive, there is no indication for treatment. If the treponemal STS result is positive and the tests are negative in a person who has not had syphilitic treatment previously, treatment is traditionally given.

Antilipid antibodies Antilipid antibodies were first detected in 1906 by Wassermann and his co-workers, who used, as antigen, extracts of liver tissue from stillborn children with congenital lues. Later it was discovered that the complement-fixing reaction was not based on the content of spirochetes in the liver, but rather on the content of lipids, and that an extract of normal tissue, for example, ox heart, could be used instead. Antilipid antibodies are not specific for the syphilitic infection, but can be found in other diseases as well. Two principles are used: the complement fixation (Wassermann) and flocculation reactions—Veneral Disease Research Laboratory test (VDRL), Kahn's reaction (KR), Meiniche's reaction (MR), Kline's test and numerous modifications.

The Rapid Plasma Reagin Card Test is suitable for quick and easy screening in the field.

Complement fixation reaction (WR) The complement fixation reaction provides a bond between antigen and antibody by the addition of an indicator system that requires complement. The indicator system consists of sheep red blood cells and anti-sheep red blood cell serum. If the patient's serum contains antilipid antibodies, these bind to the added lipid during simultaneous consumption of complement. After this, there is no complement for the indicator system's process of hemolysis.

A positive reaction is seen in the inhibition of hemolysis and titration can give a quantitative expression of the amount of antilipid antibodies. A negative reaction manifests itself in hemolysis.

Floc-culation reactions (KR and VDRL)

The flocculation reaction results can be observed with a microscope (VDRL) or directly, by macromethods (KR and MR). These results are expressed quantitatively, partly on the basis of the size of the particles and on the basis of dilution titrations.

The antilipid serum reactions normally become positive 10–14 days after appearance of the chancre. In secondary syphilis, all STS tests are strongly positive. Twenty-five percent of the patients with sero-positive primary syphilis will become negative within three months after treatment. Few will be positive after 12 months and all negative after 24 months. Secondary syphilis will revert to seronegativity within 24 months. Reinfections show a slow serological response in spite of rapid clinical improvement.

If the disease is not treated, the titer of antilipid antibodies decreases and often disappears completely. If tertiary complications develop, however, antilipid reactions often become positive again. If an otherwise sufficient treatment is begun late in the course of the disease, STS positivity may persist. This is to be regarded as a serologic scar and does not indicate a need for further treatment.

Spinal fluid examination

Late in the secondary stage, serologic study of the spinal fluid is positive in 15% of untreated patients. Examination for syphilic antibodies in the spinal fluid is indicated only in the case of suspected CNS lues and only if the serum STS is positive. A positive result is specific. If the serum STS is negative, the spinal fluid will give a negative reaction. If the serum lipid STS is positive, but the TPI is negative, a spinal tap is not indicated.

Positive treponemal tests in blood or spinal fluid do not constitute an indication for treatment if the lipid STS is negative and the patient has previously been given sufficient treatment.

Non-treponemal positive reactions

Certain diseases can lead to the formation of antilipid antibodies in patients with negative treponemal tests. This phenomenon is often called "biologic false positive" reaction; "nontreponemal" reaction, however, is the preferred term. Nontreponemal positive serum reactions are seen with collagenoses, upper respiratory tract infections, myelomatosis and leukemia. Pregnancy in healthy women can also be associated with a positive serum reaction. These reactions occur in autoimmune diseases, possibly because the antilipid reactions use tissue antigens. In syphilis, the titers of the serum reactions will normally be about the same, sometimes one of them will be positive and another "unreadable". This is seen in early syphilis, but also in nonsyphilitic illnesses accompanied by nontreponemal serum antibodies. Any unexplained positive serum reaction should be an indication for repeating the reaction, which should be supplemented by one of the antitreponemal reactions.

Treatment

Since the introduction of penicillin, treatment has resulted in cure and late manifestations of the disease no longer occur in the Northern Hemisphere.

The spirochete, in contrast to the gonococci, has apparently not changed in its sensitivity to penicillin. Since the organisms are susceptible to penicillin only during mitosis, which, as mentioned before, lasts 30 hours, the aim of treatment must be to maintain a constant serum concentration over an extended period of time. Penicillin is bactericidal, acting primarily against the cell walls of microrganisms. The spirochetes disappear from the lesion within 6–24 hours after the start of treatment.

Penicillin treatment

Early syphilis (primarily, secondary or latent less than one year) is best treated with penicillin G benzathine 2.4 million units intramuscularly given once (Half of the dose given in each gluteal region). Penicillin G procaine is an alternative given as 600,000 units given intramuscularly per day for eight days. Penicillin G benzathine in this dose will ensure an effective serum penicillin concentration for one month. The concentration in the cerebrospinal fluid will be minimal.

Late syphilis (of more than one year's duration, cardiovascular) should be treated with penicillin G procaine 600,000 units IM per day for 15 days or, as an alternative, with penicillin G benzathine 2.4 million units IM weekly for three doses.

Neurosyphilis could be treated either as late syphilis or, in order to ensure an adequate penicillin concentration, with penicillin G crystalline 2–4 million units IV every four hours for ten days.

Syphilis in pregnancy can be treated as above according to the stage, and follow-up serological tests should be performed monthly until delivery.

Congenital syphilis can occur if the mother has not received adequate treatment prior to delivery. A positive serologic test for syphilis in the newborn can be due to passive transfer of antibodies from the mother, or be due to interuterine infection. Infected infants may be asymptomatic at birth and may be sero-negative if the maternal infection occurs late in pregnancy. Children should be treated at birth if the maternal treatment was inadequate, unknown, with drugs other than penicillin, or if an adequate follow-up cannot be ensured.

It is recommended that children with congenital syphilis should have cerebrospinal examination before treatment. If the cerebrospinal fluid of the infant is normal, penicillin G benzathine 50,000 units/kg intramuscularly given once is adequate. If the cerebrospinal fluid is abnormal, treatment should aim at higher serum concentrations obtained with penicillin G crystalline, 25,000 units/kg intramuscularly or intravenously bid for at least ten days, or penicillin G procaine 50,000 units/kg intramuscularly daily for at least ten days.

Alternative treatments in case of penicillin allergy

Penicillin administration has proved to be far better than all other antisyphilitic therapeutic methods. Just as for bacterial endocarditis, penicillin treatment is such a perfect method of cure that a patient's claim of being penicillin-intolerant should be considered with skepticism and should be verified using RAST to detect any IgE serum directed against penicillin. If the result is negative, an intradermal test should be performed starting with I.U. These are somewhat unreliable tests, but if both of these examinations give negative results, they at least indicate that any reaction will not be life-threatening.

Follow-up should be performed at 3, 6 and 12 months. Retreatment should be considered if the clinical signs or syphilis persist or recur, if the titre of non-treponemal test increases, or if an initially high titre non-treponemal test fails to decrease within a year. The possibility of reinfection should always be considered. If history or tests give adequate evidence of penicillin intolerance, the following alternative medicaments are available: erythromycin, tetracycline and chloramphenicol in that order. These broad-sprectrum antibiotics are bacteriostatic interfering with DNA and RNA synthesis. In this way they influence the duplication of the microorganisms and thereby promote the host defense.

In early syphilis tetracycline or erythromycin/500 mg orally qid for 15 days is adequate. In late syphilis and neurosyphilis the same dosages are used but for 30 days. It should be noted that many patients find it difficult to remember to take four doses per day. Because of the higher dosage and the longer period of treatment, side effects and especially from the gastrointestinal tract, are quite frequent. Some patients stop treatment if diarrhea is a prominent side effect. Erythromycin should be given with meals. Tetracycline must be given one hour before or two hours after meals, since food, iron medications and some dairy products interfere with the absorption. In pregnancy tetracycline must not be used since it tends to cause staining and defects of the dentine enamel.

Gastrointestinal side effects are less frequent with chloramphenicol, which, however, is rarely used because of the risk of the blood dyscrasias.

Herxheimer's reaction This is an acute fever with simultaneous accentuation of the syphilitic lesions that begins 6–12 hours after treatment and lasts for 4–8 hours. It occurs particularly during the secondary stages but must be remembered in any treatment given for other reasons. The Herxheimer reaction is due to the spirochete death and does not indicate a penicillin intolerance. The reaction can be dangerous in older patients with cardiovascular disease. It can be prevented by oral administration of steroids (50 mg prednisolone daily) for 1–2 days before antibiotic therapy. The patient should be informed of the possibility of this febrile reaction.

Lymphogranuloma Venereum

This disease is rare. It is due to infection with a *Chlamydia,* which is closely related to that caused by TRIC agents and to psittacosis.

Clinical presentation Lymphogranuloma venereum mainly occurs and is symptomatic in men. The incubation period is not known, but in most cases it is probably less than a week. The primary lesion is a small, transitory sore, rarely seen by the physician. It can be accompanied by a transitory, indolent swelling of the lymph nodes. The most typical symptom of the disease is a marked swelling of the regional lymph nodes, with inflammation surrounding the nodes as well as above and below the inguinal ligament (the groove sign) which develops within six weeks. The nodes adhere to each other, to the underlying tissue and to the skin. The skin is bluish-red and multiple perforations develop. At this stage the patients may be ill with fever and general malaise. In women pelvic adenitis occurs, but most are seen late because of rectal stricture.

Diagnosis Previously a skin test (with lygranum antigen) was utilized, but it is no longer available on a commercial basis. Diagnosis must be based on serological tests for antibody to *Chlamydia* (compliment fixation test or microimmuno fluorescent test). Positive reactions with low titre (1:8, 1:32) can be due to previous infection with other *Chlamydia*. Patients with lymphogranuloma venereum usually have higher titres.

Therapy   The preferred therapy is sulfonamides, they produce a slow improvement even after a three week course of therapy. Penicillin is ineffective.

Chancroid

Chancroid is caused by a Gram-negative bacillus *Hemophilus ducrey,* and always sexually transmitted. It occurs in under privileged areas where hygienic conditions are poor. It has been especially common in tropical and subtropical areas, but in recent years an epidemic has swept over Greenland, which has given the opportunity of a systematic study of the disease.

Clinical features It is more frequently symptomatic in men than in women. Women have small or no symptoms although contact tracing may reveal a few minute painless ulcerations.

The incubation period is 2–7 days. In men the initial symptoms are painful small papules on the penis which develop into pustules. After destruction of the cover the pustules turn into ulcers with undermined borders and a necrotic base measuring from a few millimeters to more than a centimeter, sometimes coalescing. The most characteristic symptom is a tender swelling of a conglomerate of lymph nodes matted together above the inguinal ligament (Bubo). This lymph node swelling occurs in half of the male patients. If not treated an unilocular abscess covered by a red skin develops in which fistulae develop. Longstanding fistules with secondary autoinnoculated chancroid ulcers may eventually be the result.

Diagnosis Scrapings from the floor of the ulceration may reveal the causative agent, but the examination may fail due to secondary infection. Innoculation of pus from the ulcer onto the skin of the stomach produces a pustule within 2 or 3 days. This pustule produces a pure culture of the causative agent. An intradermal test (Ducrey) with heat-killed hemophilus bacteria will be positive several weeks after the infection, but the reaction is not diagnostic. A previously healed infection or simply a previous intradermal test with Ducrey's antigen, can result in a positive reaction.

Treatment The most reliable drugs are sulfonamides, either sulfamethoxazole 1 gram four times daily for four days, or sulfadiazine, initially four grams, followed by one gram four times daily for 10–14 days, given together with sodium bicarbonate, 1 gram four times daily and plenty of water. In case of suppuration the above mentioned treatment should be supplemented with streptomycin in a dose of one gram daily for four days. Patients who are sensitive to sulfonamide may be treated successfully with lincomycin 0.5 grams four times daily for ten days. Tetracycline has previously been recommended but has proved unsatisfactory in the present Greenland epidemic. A fluctuating bubo should always be treated by aspiration (never incision) to prevent autoinnoculation as mentioned above.

Scabies

Scabies is a frequent sexually transmitted disease. Most cases are infections acquired through intimate contact, although family and nursery epidemics occur.

The scabies mite

Scabies is caused by a 200–300-μm mite, therefore, visible by the naked eye, called *Sarcoptes scabiei*. The fertilized egg hatches after 3–4 days, after which the larvae go through one or two nymph stages and reach sexual maturity within 18 days.

Clinical presentation

The main complaint is generalized itching, especially at bedtime, when the mites' mobility increases from the warmth of the bed. The diagnosis may gain support from the patient's history (contacts who also suffer from itch). The incubation period from the time of infection until the itch begins is about 3 weeks for the first infection, but shorter for reinfections, indicating that pruritus is partly due to an allergic sensitization.

The female scabies mites tunnel the stratum corneum; in addition, burrow vesicles may be found in the adjacent (Malpighian) layer and there may be a dermal cell infiltration. The clinical picture is polymorphic; there are 4 different lesions.

1. Thread-like, dark or grayish-white burrows, 3–8-mm long, each containing 1 female mite, may be seen in most patients on the wrists or fingers, especially on the webs. The total number of burrows is usually low, since an average population of females in a patient is between 5 and 10.

2. Where the skin is thin, such as on the genitalia, the mites cause a 5–10-mm, well-defined, reddish-purple papule (Fig. 25). Such scratched papules on the

scrotum and penis of a patient whose sleep has been disturbed for several weeks by pruritus is practically pathognomonic of scabies.

3. On the trunk and upper extremities there are dispersed, scratched papulovesicles, 2–3-mm in size. These are caused by male mites, nymphs and larvae.

4. In cases of longer duration there are myriads of minimal, excoriated, punctate scratch marks, like those seen in acute spreading of an eczema ("id").

Treatment

The means of treatment are reliable against mites and nymphs, but less so against eggs. In widespread infection, therefore, it may be advisable to repeat the treatment after about 5 days, when all the eggs have hatched. Several parasiticides are available, such as gamma benzene hexachloride and crotamiton. The preparations are pleasant-smelling cream lotions that should be applied in a very thin layer over the body and the extremities, but not on the face or scalp. After 8 hours, the patient should bathe. The treatment may be repeated after 5 days if necessary.

Because of allergic senzitization, dead mites will maintain pruritus for 1 to several weeks after an otherwise succesful treatment. Sometimes scabies produces reddish-violet, intensely pruritic nodules of about 1 cm that persist for up to 1 year after treatment. These nodules are alleviated by local corticoid injections (such as triamcinolone acetonide suspension, 5 mg/ml) but sometimes excision is preferable. As with insect-bite granulomas, the historical picture may often suggest reticulosis.

Examination for other sexually transmitted diseases

Since scabies is a sexually transmitted infection, gonococci culture and STS should be performed in new patients, even if they do not have symptoms of other infections.

Pubic Lice

Etiology Phthirus pubis, pediculus pubis, or flat lice are lice that appear preferentially on the pubic hairs but which can spread to the other hairy areas, especially on the lower extremities, in the abdominal and breast areas, as well as in the axillae. In children, they are found in the eyelashes, eyebrows and margins of the scalp. The reasons for the differences in anatomical distribution are unknown. Crabs occur only in humans. The pinhead-sized brown lice sit at the base of the hairs, where they fasten themselves using the claws on their back legs. They live on blood sucked from the host. The eggs are laid at the base of the hairs and are stuck fast with chitin. After 8 days, the eggs hatch and after another 8 days the newly hatched nymphs reach sexual maturity. The life cycle is about a month; during this time, each louse lays 7–10 eggs daily.

Clinical picture After an incubation time (sensitization period), the infestation produces itchiness of an intensity that varies considerably from person to person, partly because of the differences in degrees of sensitization. Some infested persons have no pruritus, although they may have numerous crabs. As opposed to head lice, crabs less often give rise to scars from scratching or to impetigo and, therefore, do not lead to adenopathy.

At the place of the bite, where the lice inject an anticoagulant, and especially on the thigh, barely noticeable grayish-blue spots, 3–5 cm in size, develop (maculae ceruleae). Blood and feces deposits from the lice leave 0.5-cm black spots and more diffuse, blood-tinged spots on the underpants—a sign about which patients with genital pruritus should be asked specifically.

Treatment The hair in the pubic and anal regions, on the abdomen and lower extremities and perhaps in the axilla should be treated. Many insecticides are effective, but none of them necessarily penetrates the chitin shell of the egg. The treatment therefore should be repeated after 8 days, because of the hatching time, or perhaps be maintained over a period of 8 days.

The preparations used are Kwell shampoo, Kwell lotion or benzyl benzoate. Treatment with benzyl benzoate applied twice a week in the genital region and elsewhere as needed, with occasional steel combing, is recommended.

The eyelashes and eyebrows of children can be treated with petrolatum.

Condylomata Acuminata

Condylomata acuminata, or genital warts, are papillomatous, cauliflower-like tumors in the anogenital region, on the mucous membrane and the surrounding skin.

Etiology Condyloma acuminatum is due to a papovavirus that is related to but not proved identical with verruca vulgaris virus. The virus cannot be cultured, but can be isolated and inoculated. Histologic examination reveals hyperkeratosis, parakeratosis and acanthosis, as well as inclusion bodies.

Epedimiology The age distribution is identical with that of gonorrhea, suggesting that this also is a sexually transmitted disease.

An examination of partners of English soldiers who had been infected with condylomas in Malaysia showed that in two thirds, lesions developed within 3 months; the incubation period, however, can be longer.

Anal condylomata occur especially in patients who had anal intercourse, but since the contacts are often found to be asymptomatic, it is assumed that the virus can occur in the gastrointestinal tract and be inoculated through trauma.

Warts on the hand are not relevant as a cause of infection, just as warts on the fingers do not occur after handling condylomata.

Clinical presentation Condylomata are white or pink papillomas of small size initially, which develop a lobulated surface as they grow. In spite of the abundant vascularization, they have no tendency to bleed during intercourse and the symptoms are minimal, often only cosmetic.

In men, condylomata acuminata are localized on the inner side of the prepuce, especially on the coronal sulcus and around the frenulum (Fig. 29). In the rare cases of localization on the glans, the condylomata have a flat base. In about one third of male patients, condylomata are found in the urethral meatus (Fig. 30). These are resistant to treatment and often require referral to a specialist. Condylomata on the skin are less lobulated and may resemble ordinary warts. Anal condylomata occur equally often in men and women (Fig. 31).

In women, condylomata are most frequent on the inner side of the labiae minorae and the posterior commissure, the perineum, perianal area and in the posterior part of the vagina. They sometimes occur on the labiae majorae, in the vagina, on the cervix and on the skin. Intraurethral condylomata are infrequent in women. In pregnant women and those using oral contraceptives, condylomata have a tendency to spread and grow quickly. In the latter half of pregnancy, their growth can be explosive. They do not hinder giving birth, however, and do not infect the infant. Such children may develop laryngeal papylomatosis. Perianal condylomata occur in small children, but otherwise they are rare in childhood in contrast to warts.

Treatment Podophyllin is used in a 10–20% alcohol solution or in tincture of benzoin, which is painted on the warts with a cotton swab; the superfluous solution is dried off. It is helpful to place cotton or gauze under the prepuce, in the vulva or anal region to avoid contact of the solution with the normal skin. The solution should be washed off after 4–8 hours, using soap and water. The treatment is repeated weekly, until the condylomata disappear or until surgical excision is undertaken.

The medication should rarely be given for home use, since the protracted course of the disease will tempt to overtreatment and secondary ulcerations may result. Normally, the treatment must be repeated several times.

Treatment during pregnancy is often useless and should be postponed until after delivery. If used over extended surfaces Podophyllin may cause abortions. Fluorouracil used daily for 3–4 weeks is approximately as efficient as Podophyllin. Until Podophyllin was introduced, treatment was by surgery; if Podophyllin treatment proves ineffective, curettage under local anesthesia is considered. This applies especially to intraurethral or perianal condylomas; if conservative Podophyllin treatment has not cured within a relatively short period, surgical treatment is preferred. For intraurethral condylomas, a Lidocaine gel is an effective local anesthetic. Curettage is preferable to electrodesiccation to avoid scarring.

Supplementary examination

Patients with condylomata should be examined for other venereal diseases, especially gonorrhea, during the first consultation. Women must be examined for *Trichomonas vaginalis,* since maceration combined with secretion promotes growth of condyloma.

Differential diagnoses

The most important differential diagnosis is syphilitic papules, which are flat, broad-based and macerated (condylomata lata). These are revealed by a dark-field examination at the first visit or by a positive STS.

In men, pearly penile papules, small papules on the corona, can be mistaken for condylomata. The papules are uniformly large, however, and lack the tumor-like appearance of condylomata. The patient will often state that they have been present for years. These require no treatment.

Molluscum Contagiosum

Molluscum contagiosum is characterized by dome-shaped, white or yellowish lesions up to 5 mm in size, which have a slight central depression (umbilical formation). The lesions are produced by a pox virus. The incubation time is between 3 weeks and 3 months.

Epidemiology Infection can occur at swimming pools, in steam baths, but also by intimate contact in wrestling, playing or during intercourse. The localization of sexually transmitted molluscum is around the genital area, on the abdomen and thighs. In homosexuals, the lesions will be observable on the buttocks. The infection produces no symptoms unless secondary infection occurs.

Treatment The lesions are punctured with a pointed scalpel, after which a small, firm, white grain can be squeezed out. Curettage after ethyl chloride freezing can also be used.

Balanitis

Balanitis, or balanoposthitis, is a surface inflammation located on the glans and foreskin. It occurs especially often in men with a long, tight foreskin.

Etiology Balanitis can be caused by *Candida albicans, Trichomonas, Herpes virus* or various bacteria, but can also be an expression of contact dermatitis. Poor hygiene facilitates its development. All patients with balanitis should be tested for diabetes.

Symptoms The symptoms are diffuse redness of the glans extending over the inner surface of the prepuce, sometimes with exudation that may be abundant and purulent. The patient complains of pruritus and stinging. There can be well-defined surface erosions or a well-defined erythema. Often there is only a moderate exudate; characteristically, however, there is no urethral discharge.

Treatment Before the result of bacteriologic or mycologic test is available, it would be advisable to use a cortocoid-combination preparation that has an anti-inflammatory and antimicrobial effect. This treatment should not be given for an extended period because of risk of cortocoid atrophy. Any topical treatment can produce a proliferating hyperkeratosis that may be misinterpreted as continued illness. Such a hyperkeratosis is cured by wet compresses.

A water compress, possibly with a mild antiseptic, changed several times daily, will frequently be the only treatment effecting a cure. If a tight and not retractable prepuce is present, treatment should begin by rinsing the preputial space with an antimicrobial solution in a disposable syringe, repeated several times daily. This may calm the inflammation enough for the foreskin to be retracted. Diagnostically, be aware that a carcinoma can produce balanitis and continued recurrence should be treated by circumcision. A chancre can also hide behind a tight foreskin.

Synergistic Gangrene

This is an extremely rare disease which, just like any synergistic gangrene of the skin, can develop in the course of several days and cause significant loss of tissue in the glans and the upper part of the penis. The cause is unknown. The illness is quickly cured by antibiotic treatment, but may result in considerable loss of tissue.

Hepatitis

In secondary syphilis a complicatius hepatitis with negative Australia antigen test disappears with adequate treatment with penicillin. Routine screening with Australia antigen (HBAG) reveals a number of symptom free carriers among promiscuous persons, especially homosexual men, where the incidence is four times higher than that found among heterosexual males. Risk groups for hepatitis B are beside homosexual males, prostitutes, drug abusers, tattooed persons and persons with previous liver disease.

Women may develop a gonorrheic perihepatitis, which starts with pain in the right upper abdominal quadrant with fever, tenderness and pain at inspiration. Culture from the genitals will show gonococci.

Other Skin Diseases of the Genitalia

Some of the skin diseases that can manifest themselves on the genital mucous membranes of both sexes include psoriasis (Fig. 35), lichen planus (Fig. 36) and uncommon forms of fixed drug eruptions. In men, a precancerous disease, Bowen's disease of the skin, can also occur.

Venerophobia

Groundless, persistent fear of having contracted a sexually transmitted disease occurs almost exclusively in men. The anxiety can be traced either to a past illness or simply to having been exposed to contagion in a suspect relationship.

Persons who present with these complaints should be given a complete venerologic examination and are entitled to a painstaking explanation of the symptomatology of venereal diseases and especially of the extremely benign prognosis associated with correctly administered treatment. An all too extended follow-up period after correct treatment may have contributed to the patient's anxiety.

On the other hand, it must be remembered that many persons have previously had a diagnosis of venerophobia because they were suffering from a non-gonorrheic urethritis that went unrecognized after tests for gonococci were performed and proved to be negative.

Plates

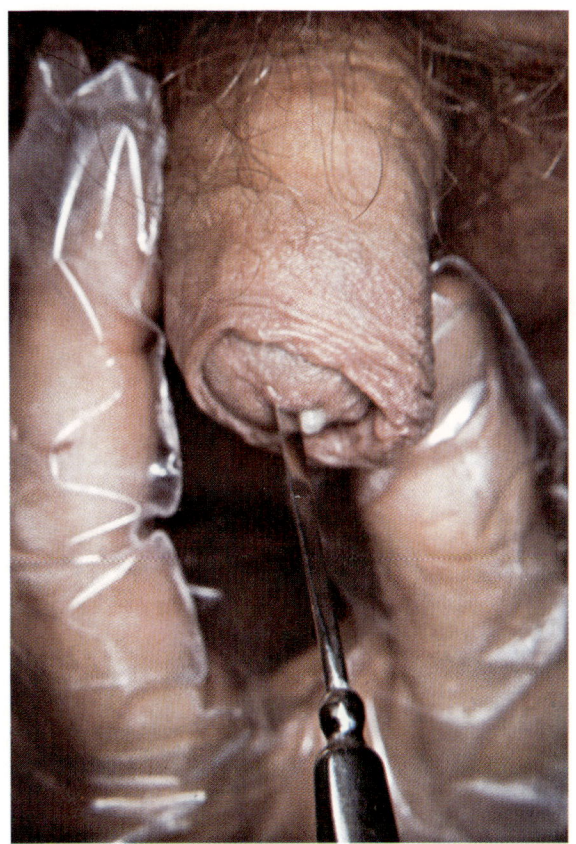

Fig. 1. Urethral sampling.

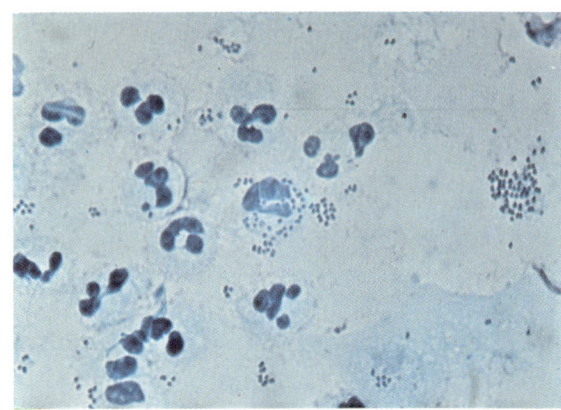

Fig. 2. Urethral secretion from a male stained with methylene blue. Note the intracellular and extracellular diplococci.

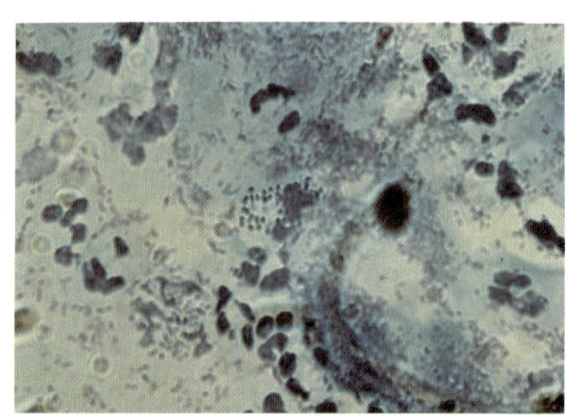

Fig. 3. Methylene blue stain smear of cervical discharge in gonorrhea.

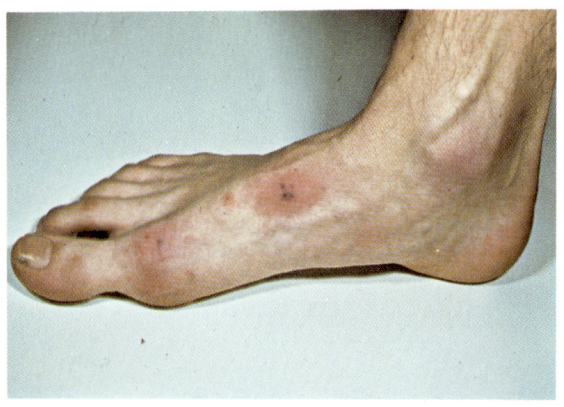

Fig. 4. Pustules on the foot in gonorrhea-arthritis-dermatitis syndrome.

Fig. 5. Pustules on the hand in gonorrhea-arthritis-dermatitis syndrome.

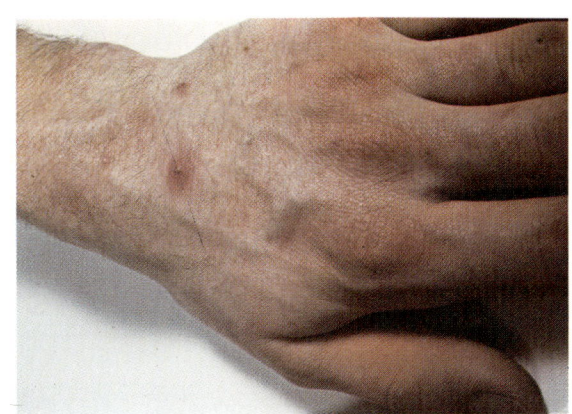

Fig. 6. Large, round blastlike cells with strongly colored nuclei in nongonorrheal urethritis.

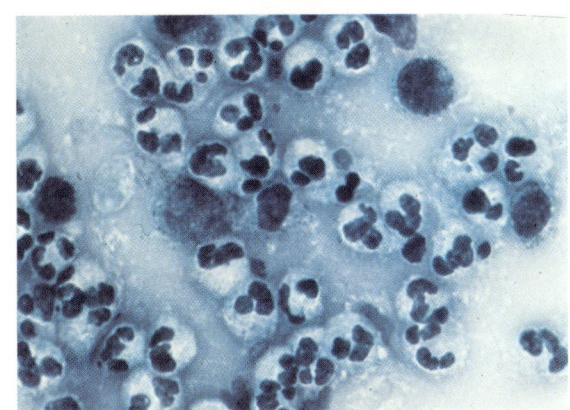

Fig. 7. Inclusion bodies in large mononuclear cells as seen after Giemsa staining.

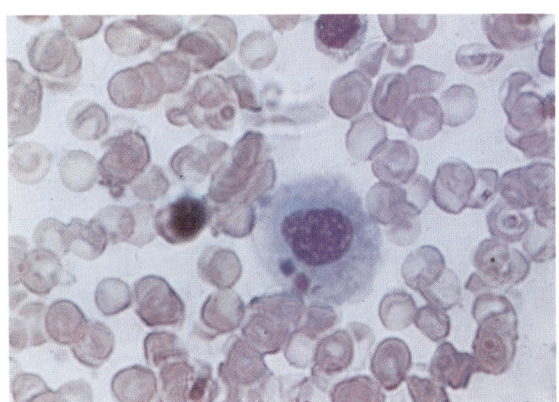

Fig. 8. Circinate balanitis in Reiter's syndrome.

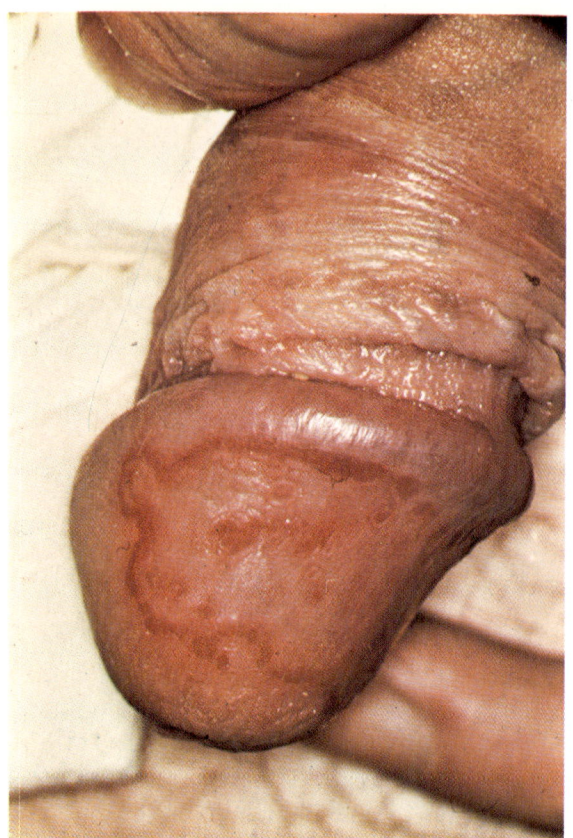

Fig. 9. Candida balanitis.

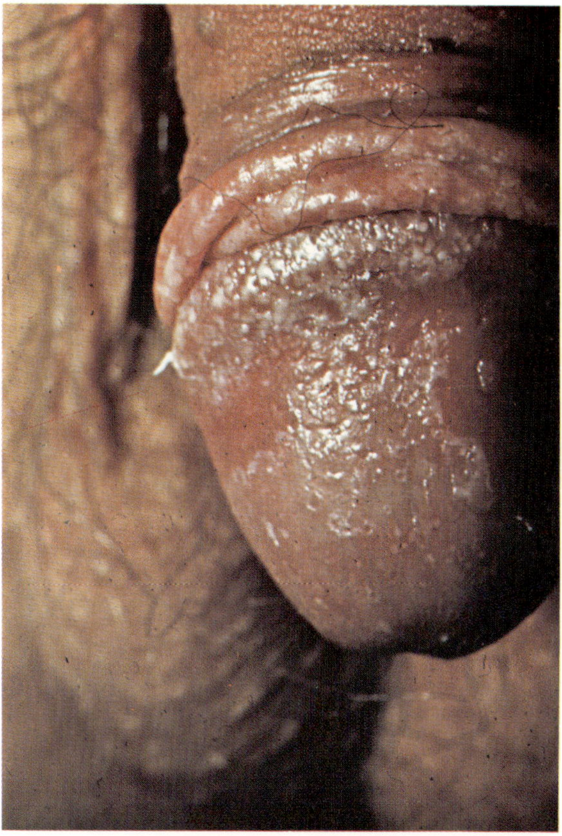

Fig. 10. Herpes simplex on the areola.

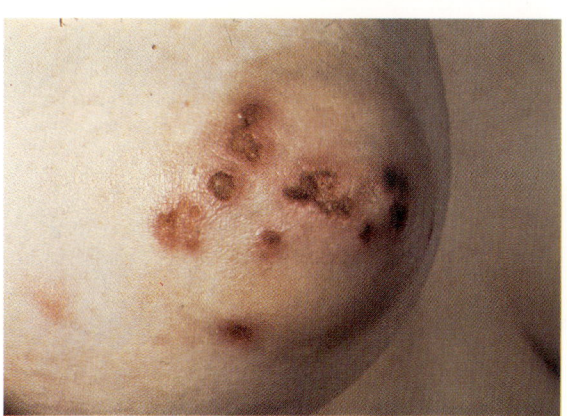

Fig. 11. Herpes progenitalis.

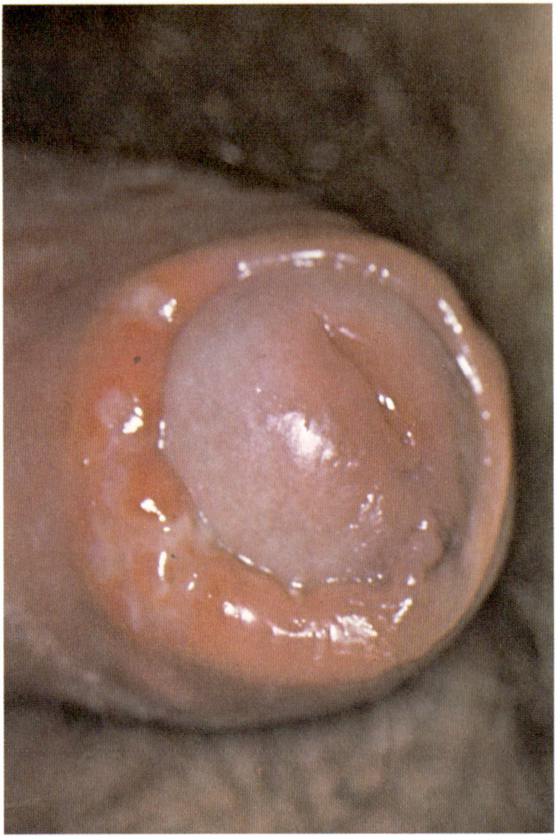

Fig. 12. Scraping of the base of a herpes simplex vesicle showing multinucleated giant cells.

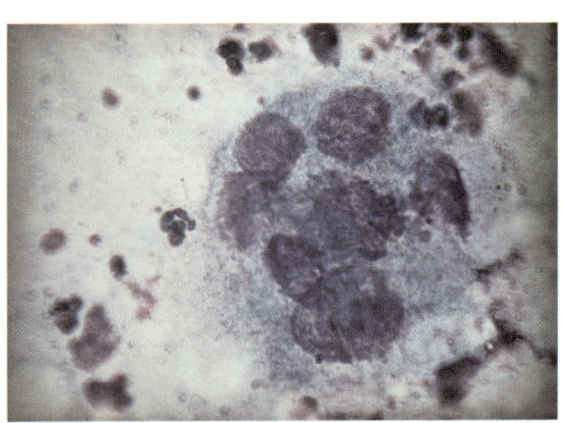

Fig. 13. Preputial syphylitic chancre.

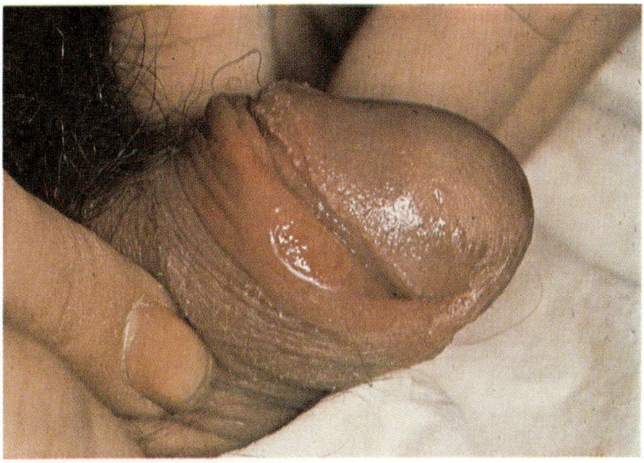

Fig. 14. Syphylitic chancre.

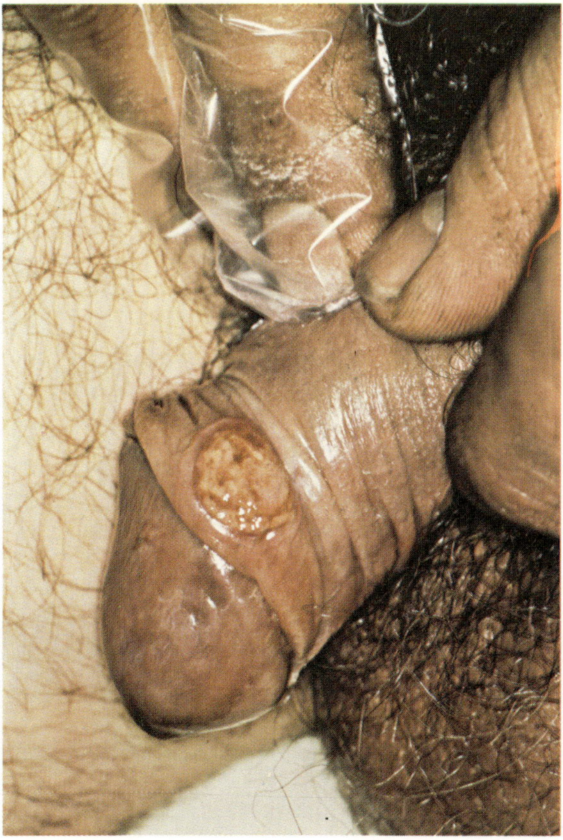

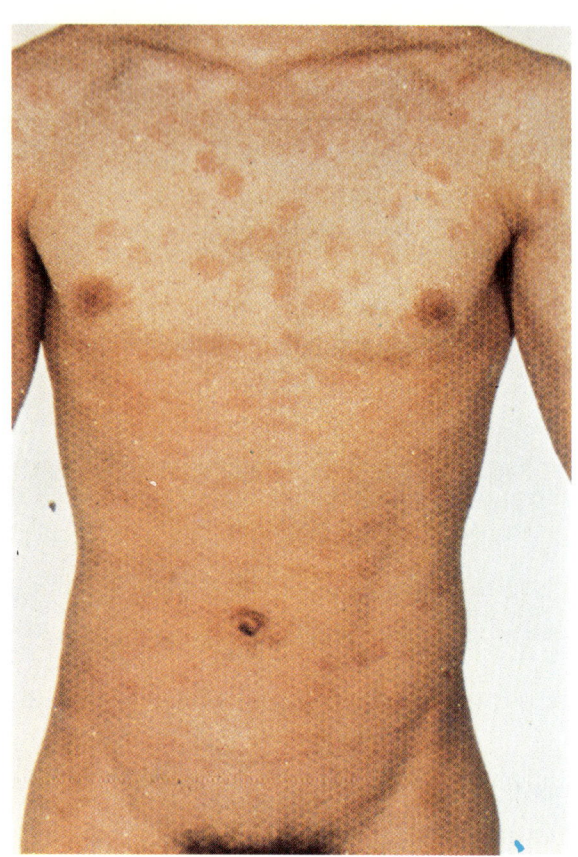

Fig. 15. Roseola.

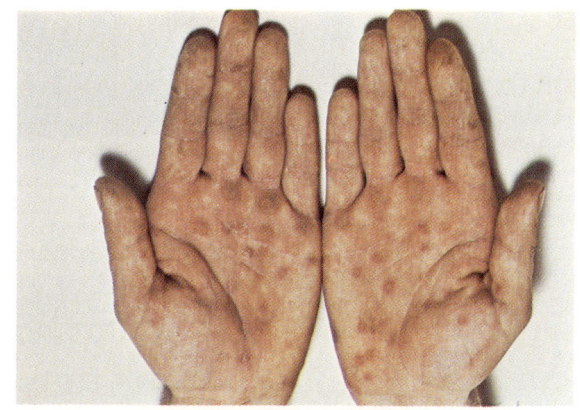

Fig. 16. Palmar papules in secondary syphilis.

Fig. 17. Plantar papules in secondary syphilis.

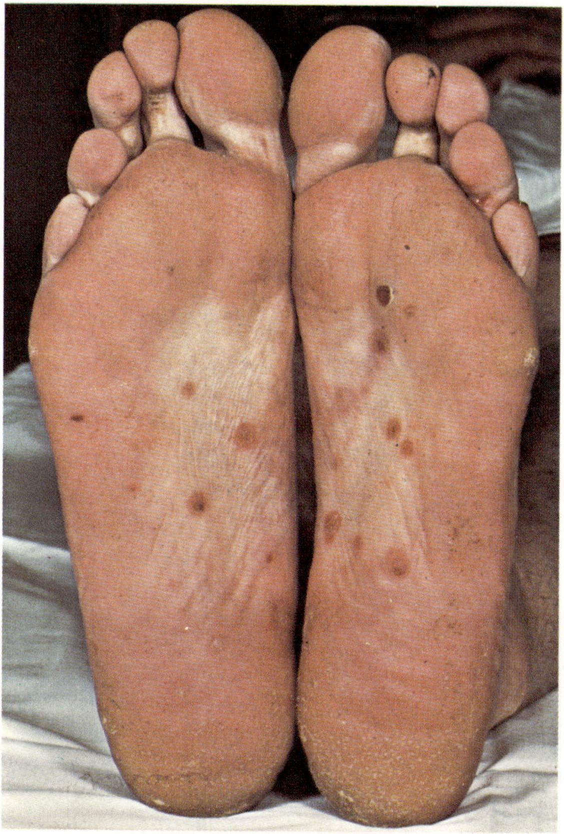

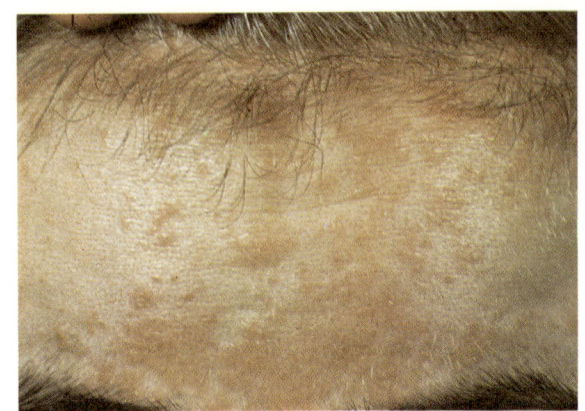

Fig. 18. Seborrheic-like luetic papules on the forehead.

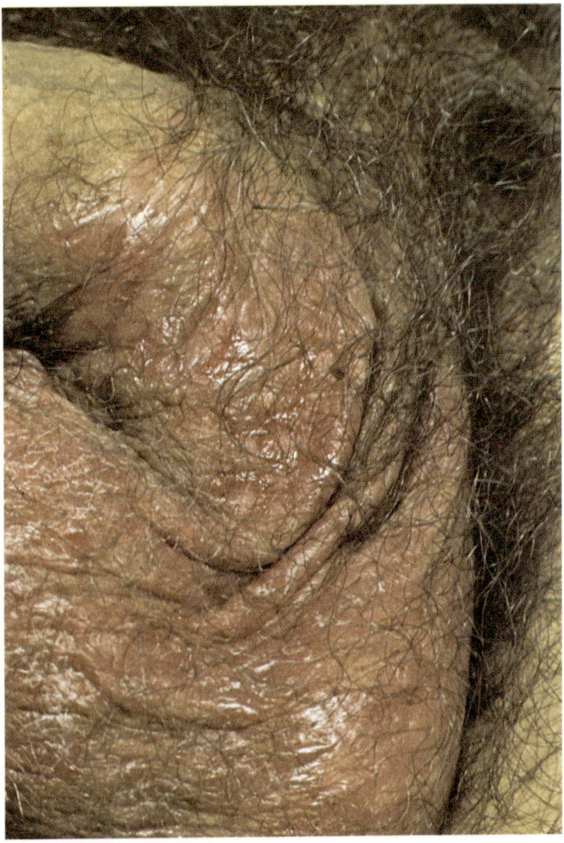

Fig. 19. Eroded genital papules in secondary syphilis.

Fig. 20. Circumoral seborrheic-like papules in secondary syphilis.

Fig. 21. Secondary syphilitic papules on the posterior commissure.

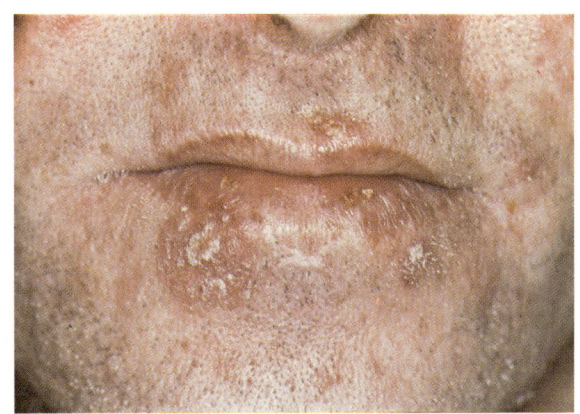

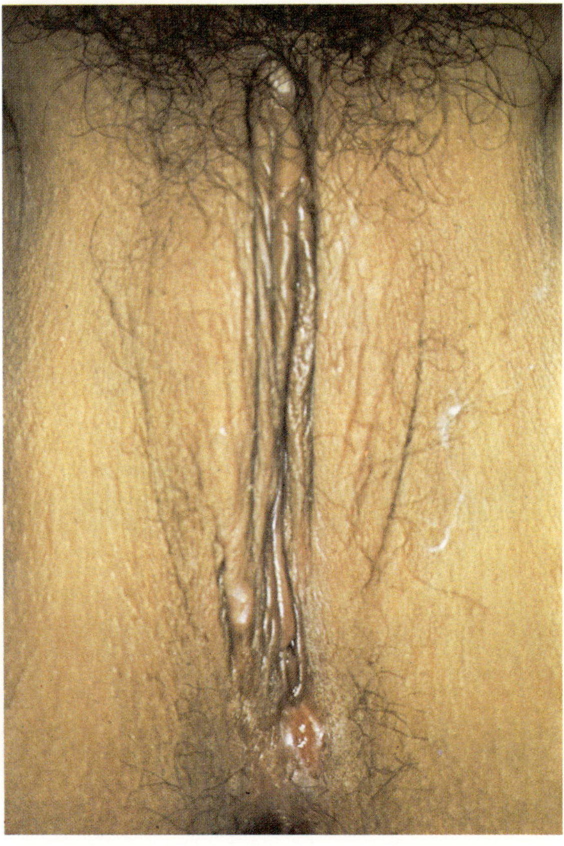

Fig. 22. Anal papules in secondary syphilis.

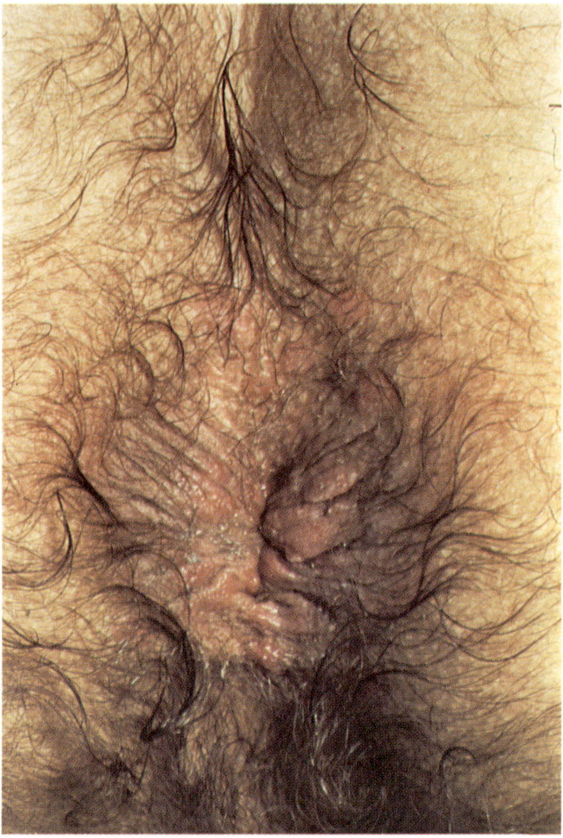

Fig. 23. Tongue papules–secondary syphilis.

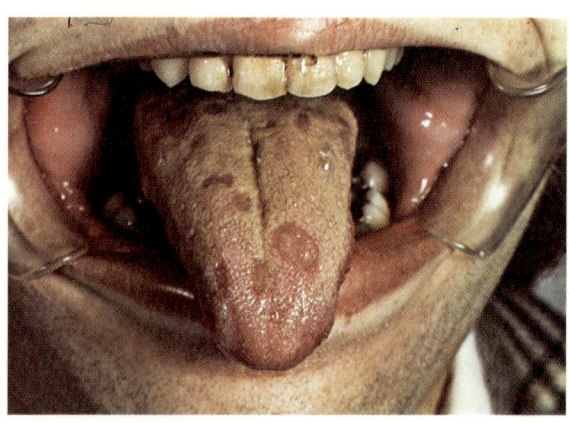

Fig. 24. Palatal papules– secondary syphilis.

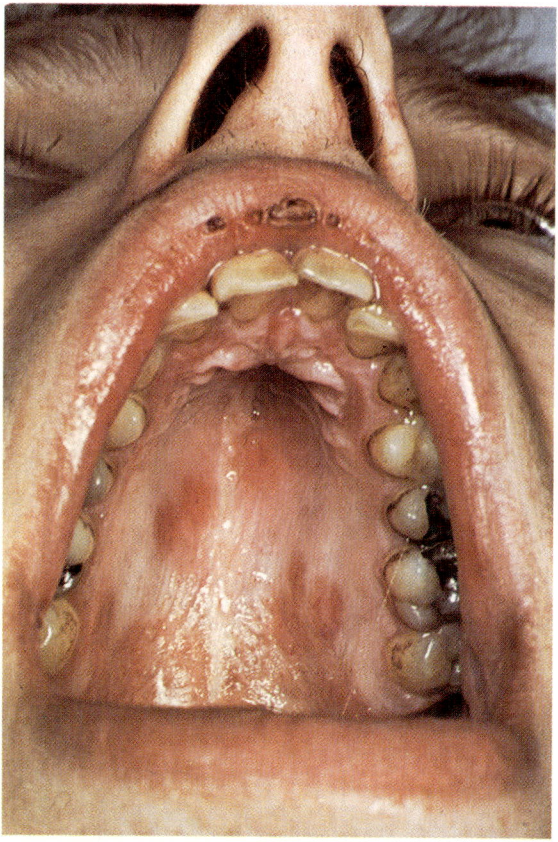

Fig. 25. Scabietic papules on the genitals and surrounding area.

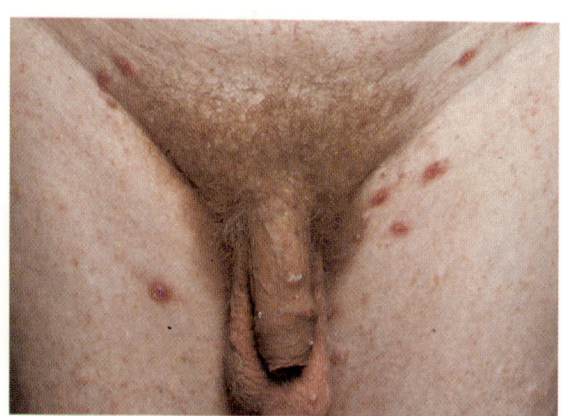

Fig. 26. Pubic louse.

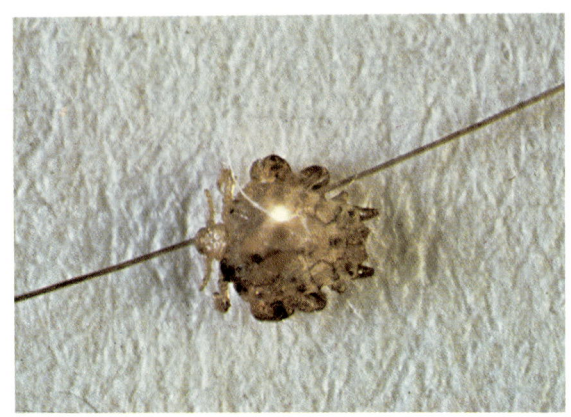

Fig. 27. Pubic lice.

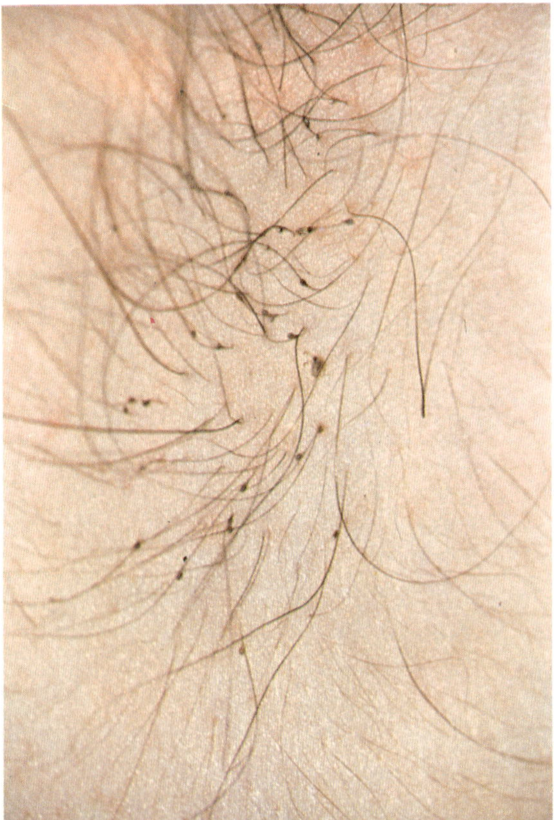

Fig. 28. Pubic lice on cilia.

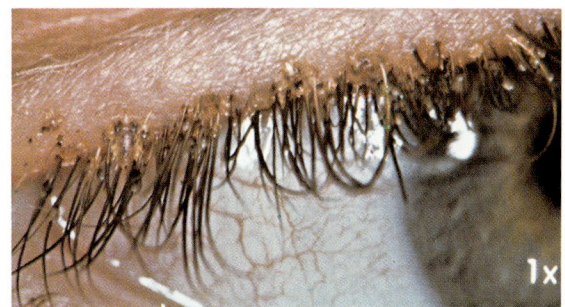

Fig. 29. Venereal warts.

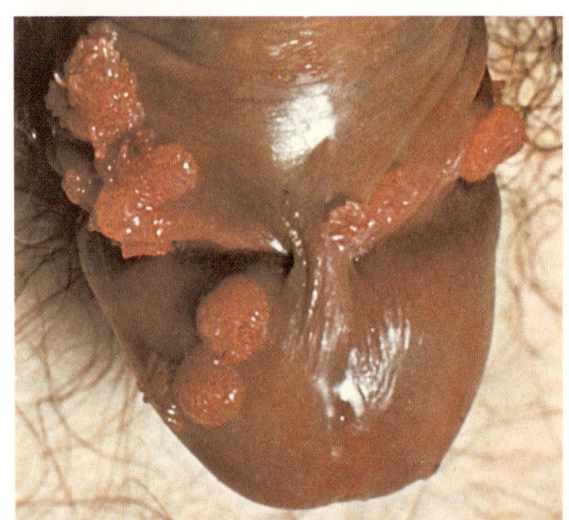

Fig. 30. Condylomata acuminata– intraurethral.

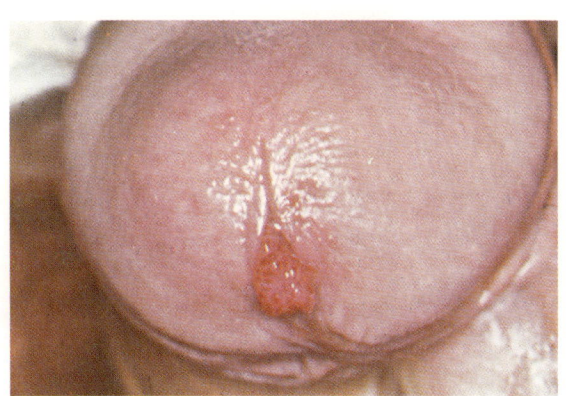

Fig. 31. Condylomata acuminata–anal.

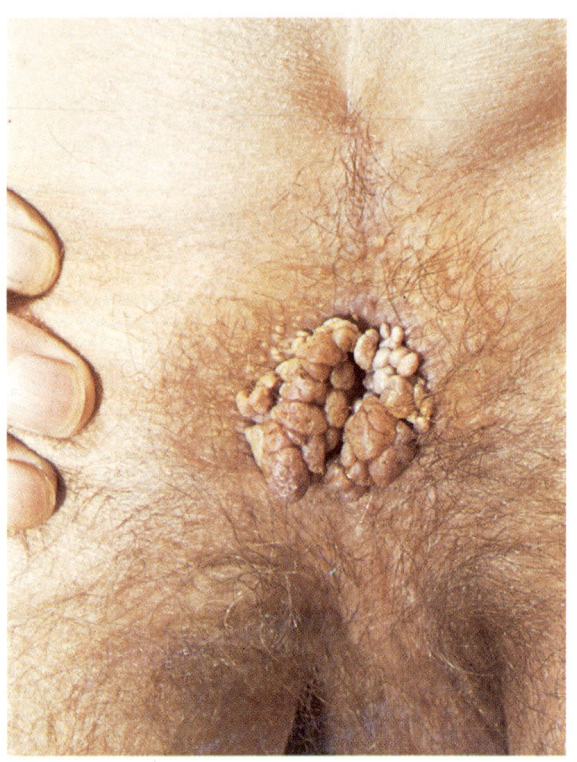

Fig. 32. Pearly penile papules that do not represent venereal disease.

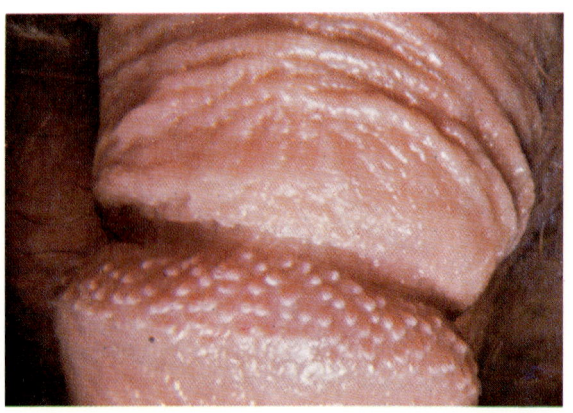

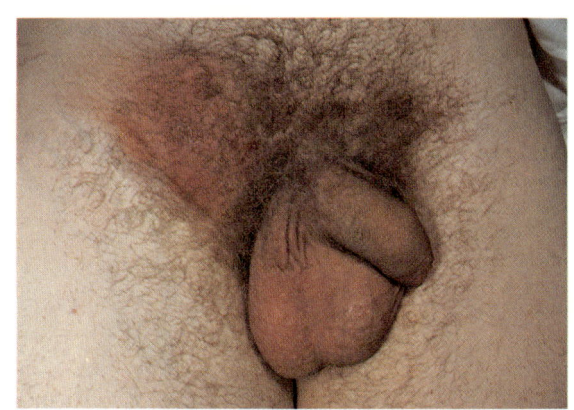

Fig. 33. Bubo in connection with chancroid.

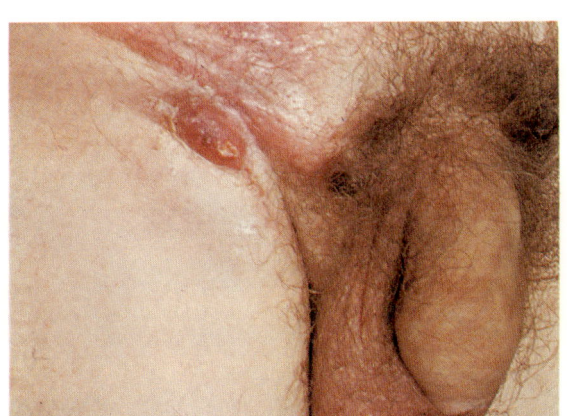

Fig. 34. Lymphadenopathy as seen in L.G.V. with the characteristic groove sign.

Fig. 35. Psoriasis–glans.

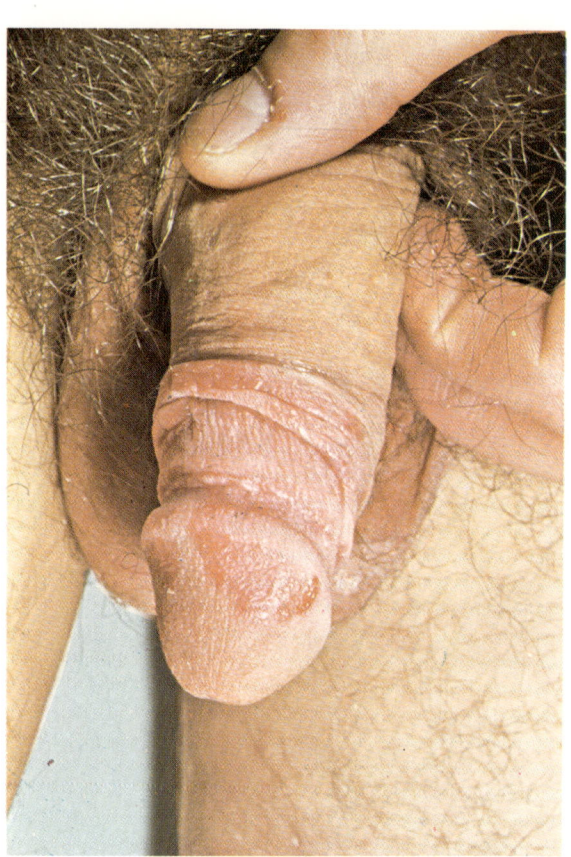

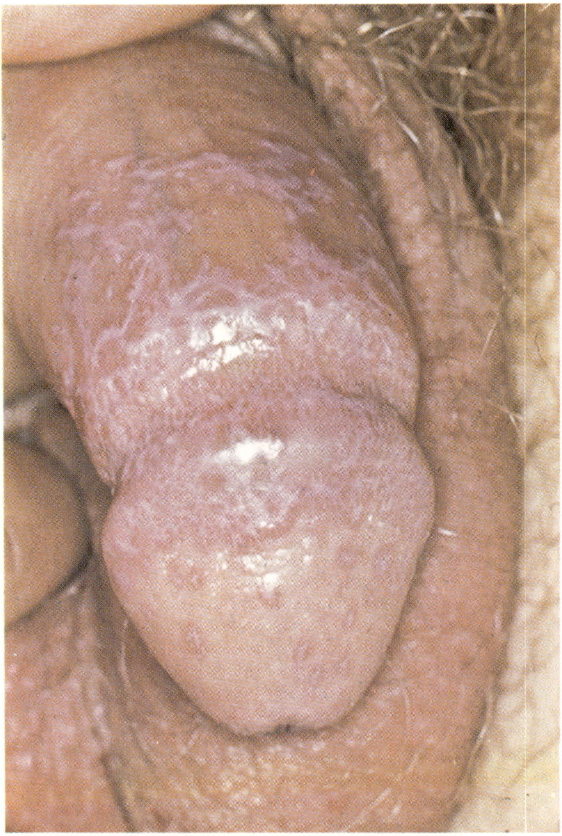

Fig. 36. Lichen planus.

Fig. 37. Lichen sclerosus et atrophicus with phimosis.

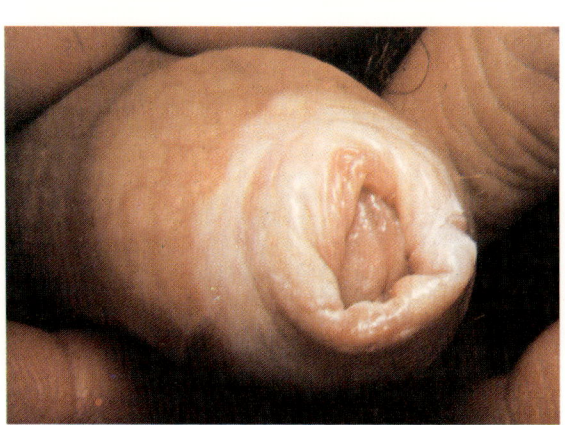

Fig. 38. Lichen sclerosus et atrophicus–vulva.

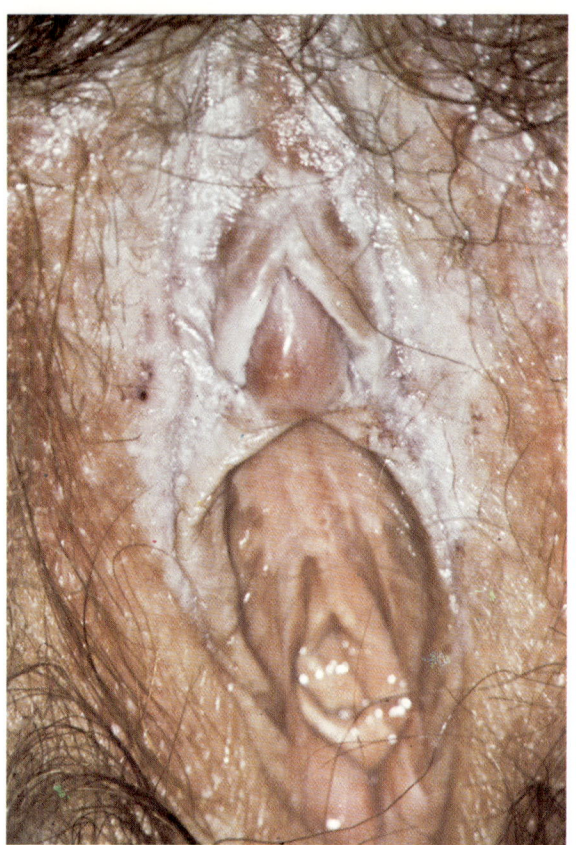

Fig. 39. Erythroplasia of Queyrat.

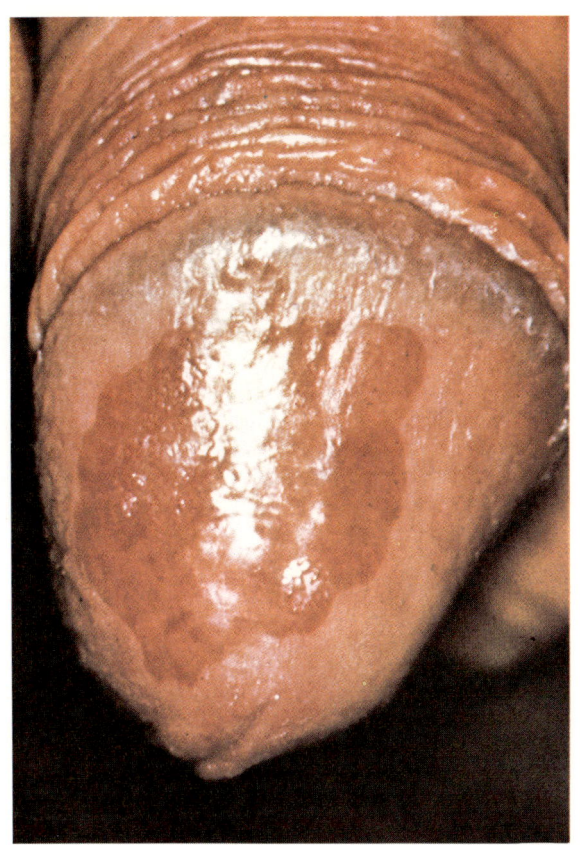

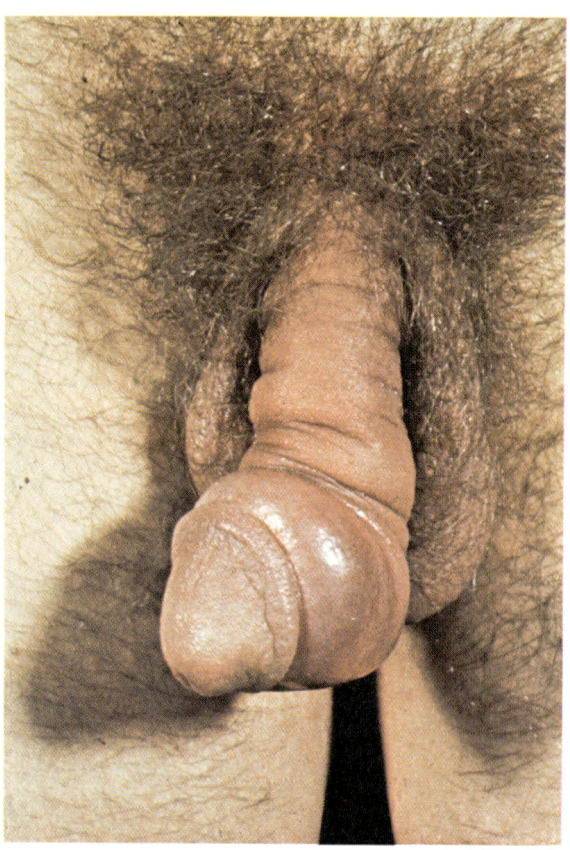

Fig. 40. Preputial edema with paraphimosis.

Index

A

Allergy: to penicillin in syphilis, alternative treatments, 54–55
Anal
  condylomata acuminata, 92
  examination, 9
  papules in secondary syphilis, 88
Antibiotics: resistance of gonococci to, 23
Antibodies
  antilipid, in syphilis, 50
  treponemal, 49
Antilipid antibodies: in syphilis, 50
Areola: herpes simplex on, 81
Arthritis
  -dermatitis syndrome, 15–16
  -gonorrhea-dermatitis syndrome, 78–79
  monarthritis, gonorrheic, 16

B

Bacterial nongonorrheic urethritis, 30
Balanitis, 69–70
  Candida, 81
  circinate, in Reiter's syndrome, 80
  etiology, 69
  symptoms, 69
  treatment, 69–70
Bartholinitis, 15
Blastlike cells: in nongonorrheal urethritis, 79
Bubo: and chancroid, 93

C

Candida
  balanitis, 81
  urethritis, 36
Candidiasis, 36–37
  clinical presentation, 36–37
  treatment, 37

Cells
  blastlike, in nongonorrheal urethritis, 79
  giant, multinucleated, in herpes simplex vesicle, 82
  mononuclear, in inclusion bodies, 79
Cervical discharge smear: in gonorrhea, with methylene blue stain, 78
Cervicitis, 14
Chancres
  extragenital, 44
  syphilis, 83
Chancroid, 59
  bubo and, 93
  clinical presentation, 59
  treatment, 60
Check-up, 10
Cilia: pubic lice on, 91
Circinate balanitis: in Reiter's syndrome, 80
Circumoral seborrheic-like papules: in secondary syphilis, 87
Commissure: posterior, secondary syphilitic papules on, 87
Complement fixation reaction: in syphilis, 50
Condylomata acuminata, 65–67
  anal, 92
  clinical presentation, 65–66
  diagnosis, differential, 67
  epidemiology, 65
  etiology, 65
  examination for other venereal diseases in, 67
  intraurethral, 91
  supplementary examination in, 67
  treatment, 66–67
Congenital syphilis, 46
Conjunctival TRIC infections, 27–29
Contamination: in venereal disease, tracing source of, 7
Culture in gonorrhea, 18–19
  medium for, 20
Cystitis, 13

D

Definition: of venereal disease, 5
Dermatitis
  -arthritis-syndrome, 15–16

-gonorrhea-arthritis syndrome, 78–79
Diplococci: intracellular and extracellular, 78

E

Edema: preputial, with paraphimosis, 98
Epidemiology
   in condylomata acuminata, 65
   in molluscum contagiosum, 68
   in trichomoniasis, 34
Epididymitis, 13
Erythroplasia of Queyrat, 97
Etiology
   in balanitis, 69
   in condylomata acuminata, 65
   of pubic lice, 63
Examination, 8–10
   anal, 9
   genital, 8
   of men, 8–9
   microscopic, in gonorrhea, 18
   oral cavity, 9
   spinal fluid, in syphilis, 51
   of women, 9–10
Experimental infection: in gonorrhea, 11

F

Flocculation reactions: in syphilis, 50
Fluor vaginalis, 14
Follow-up in gonorrhea, 25
   serologic, 25
Foot pustules: in gonorrhea-arthritis-dermatitis syndrome, 78
Forehead: seborrheic-like luetic papules on, 86
FTA test: in syphilis, 46

G

Gangrene: synergistic, 71
Genital
   examination, 8
   papules
     eroded, in secondary syphilis, 86
     scabietic, 89
   skin diseases, 73
   TRIC infections, 27

Giant cells: multinucleated, in herpes simplex vesicle, 82
Giemsa stain: of inclusion bodies in mononuclear cells, 79
Glans: psoriasis, 94
Gonococci, 11
  resistance to antibiotics, 23–24
Gonorrhea, 11–25
  -arthritis-dermatitis syndrome, 78–79
  asymptomatic, 12
  cervical discharge smear with methylene blue stain, 78
  culture in, 18–19
    medium, 20
  diagnosis, 17–20
  experimental infection, 11
  extragenital, 15–17
  follow-up, 25
    serologic, 25
  immunity in, 11
  incubation time, 11
  inoculation in, 19
  intercourse ban, 24–25
  in men, 12–13
    diagnosis, incorrect, 13
    symptom duration, 12
    symptomatic infections, weakly, 12
  microscopic examination in, 18
  oral therapy in, 21–22
  parenteral therapy in, 21
  preparation staining in, 17–18
  prognosis, 25
  resistance to
    determination of, 20
    pattern of, 24
  sampling in, 17
  tonsil, 15
  transport substrate, 20
  treatment, 21–25
  in women, 13–15
Gonorrheic monarthritis, 16
Groove sign: in lymphadenopathy in lymphogranuloma venereum, 93

H

Hand pustules: in gonorrhea-arthritis-dermatitis syndrome, 73
Herpes
  genitalis urethritis, 38
  progenitalis, 38–41, 78
    clinical presentation, 38–39
    diagnosis, 39–40
    treatment, 40–41
  simplex
    on areola, 81
    vesicle with multinucleated giant cells, 82
Herxheimer's reaction: and syphilis treatment, 55–56
History: of syphilis, 42

I

Immunity: in gonorrhea, 11
Incidence: of venereal disease, 5–6
Inclusion bodies: in mononuclear cells, 79
Incubation time: in gonorrhea, 11–12
Inoculation: in gonorrhea, 19
Intercourse ban, 10
  in gonorrhea, 24–25
Intraurethral condylomata acuminata, 91

K

KR: in syphilis, 51

L

Lice, pubic, 63–64, 90
  on cilia, 91
  clinical picture in, 63
  etiology, 63
  treatment, 64
Lichen planus, 95
Lichen sclerosus et atrophicus
  phimosis and, 95
  on vulva, 96
Luetic papules: on forehead, 86
Lymphadenopathy: in lymphogranuloma venereum, 93
Lymphogranuloma venereum, 57–58

clinical presentation, 57
lymphadenopathy in, 87
treatment, 53

M

Men
  examination of, 8–9
  gonorrhea in (*see* Gonorrhea, in men)
  urethral secretion from, with methylene blue stain, 78
Methylene blue stain
  of cervical discharge smear in gonorrhea, 78
  of urethral secretion in male, 78
Microscopic diagnosis: of syphilis, 48
Mite: of scabies, 61
Molluscum contagiosum, 68
  epidemiology, 68
  treatment, 68
Monarthritis: gonorrheic, 16
Mononuclear cells: inclusion bodies in, 79
Multinucleated giant cells: in herpes simplex vesicle, 82
Mycoplasma, 29

O

Ophthalmoblenorrhea, 16
Oral
  cavity, examination of, 9
  therapy, in gonorrhea, 21–22

P

Palatal papules: in secondary syphilis, 89
Palmar papules: in secondary syphilis, 85
Papules
  penile, not a venereal disease, 92
  scabietic, on genitals, 89
  seborrheic-like
    circumoral, in secondary syphilis, 87
    luetic, on forehead, 86
  in secondary syphilis (*see* Syphilis, secondary, papules in)
Paraphimosis: and preputial edema, 98
Parenteral therapy: in gonorrhea, 21

Penicillin
  allergy in syphilis, alternative treatments, 54–55
  deposit, in syphilis, 53
Penile papules: not a venereal disease, 92
Phimosis
  lichen sclerosus et atrophicus and, 95
  paraphimosis and preputial edema, 98
Plantar papules: in secondary syphilis, 85
Pregnant patients with syphilis: treatment of, 47
Preputial
  edema with paraphimosis, 98
  syphylitic chancre, 83
Proctitis, 13, 15
Prostatitis, 13
Psoriasis: glans, 94
Pubic lice (*see* Lice, pubic)
Pustules in gonorrhea-arthritis-dermatitis syndrome
  on foot, 78
  on hand, 79

Q

Queyrat erythroplasia, 97

R

Reiter's syndrome, 32–33
  balanitis in, circinate, 80
  treatment, 31
Resistance
  of gonococci to antibiotics, 23
  to gonorrhea, determination of, 20
  pattern in gonorrhea, 24
Roseola, 84

S

Salpingitis, 14
Sampling
  in gonorrhea, 17
  urethral, 87
Scabies, 61–62
  clinical presentation, 61–62
  examination for other venereal diseases in, 62
  genital papules in, 89

mite, 61
treatment, 62
Seborrheic-like papules (*see* Papules, seborrheic-like)
Serologic diagnosis: of syphilis, 49
Sexually committed diseases (*see* Venereal disease)
Skin diseases: of genitalia, 66
Spinal fluid examination: in syphilis, 51
Spirochaeta pallida, 42
Synergistic gangrene, 71
Syphilis, 42–47
  antilipid antibodies in, 50
  chancre, 83
    preputial, 83
  clinical features, 43–47
  complement fixation reaction in, 50
  congenital, 46
  diagnosis
    microscopic, 48
    serologic, 49
  etiology, 42–43
  extragenital chancres, 44
  flocculation reactions in, 51
  FTA test in, 49
  Herxheimer's reaction and, 55
  history, 42
  KR in, 51
  latent, 45
  masked, 23
  nontreponemal positive reactions in, 52
  penicillin allergy in, alternative treatments, 54–55
  penicillin in, deposit, 53
  primary ulceration, 43
  secondary, 44–45
  secondary, papules in
    anal, 88
    circumoral seborrheic-like, 87
    genital, eroded, 86
    palatal, 89
    palmar, 85
    plantar, 85
    on posterior commissure, 87
    tongue, 88

spinal fluid examination in, 51
tertiary, 45–46
TPI in, 49
treatment, 53–54
  of pregnant patients, 47
treponemal antibodies in, 49
VDRL in, 51
WR in, 50

T

Tongue papules: in secondary syphilis, 88
Tonsil gonorrhea, 15
TPI: in syphilis, 49
Treatment procedure: for venereal disease, 6
Treponema pallidum, 42
Treponemal antibodies, 49
TRIC agents, 27
Trichomonas urethritis, 31
Trichomoniasis, 34–35
  clinical presentation, 34
  detection, 35
  epidemiology, 34
  treatment, 35

U

Ulceration: primary, in syphilis, 43
Urethra
  condylomata acuminata of, 91
  sampling, 77
  secretion from male with methylene blue stain, 78
Urethritis, 14
  bacterial nongonorrheic, 30
  Candida, 36
  herpes genitalis, 38
  nongonococcal, 26
    round blastlike cells with colored nuclei in, 79
    treatment, 29
  trichomonas, 34

V

Vaginalis: fluor, 14
Vaginitis: vulvovaginitis, 17
VDRL: in syphilis, 51

Venereal disease
  contamination, tracing source of, 7
  definition, 5
  examination for (*see* Examination)
  incidence, 5–6
  treatment procedure, 6
Venereal warts, 91
Venereology (*see* Venereal disease)
Venerophobia, 74
Vesicle: of herpes simplex, with multinucleated giant cells, 82
Vulva: lichen sclerosus et atrophicus on, 96
Vulvovaginitis, 17

W

Warts: venereal, 91
Women
  examination of, 9–10
  gonorrhea in, 13–15
WR: in syphilis, 50